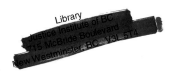
Cool
Connections
with **Cognitive**
Behavioural
Therapy

of related interest

Helping Children to Build Self-Esteem
A Photocopiable Activities Book
2nd edition
Deborah Plummer
Illustrated by Alice Harper
ISBN 978 1 84310 488 9

Self-Esteem Games for Children
Deborah Plummer
Illustrated by Jane Serrurier
ISBN 978 1 84310 424 7

No More Stinking Thinking
A Workbook for Teaching Children Positive Thinking
Joann Altiero
ISBN 978 1 84310 839 9

Special Stories for Disability Awareness
Stories and Activities for Teachers, Parents and Professionals
Mal Leicester
Illustrated by Taryn Shrigley-Wightman
ISBN 978 1 84310 390 5

Classroom Tales
Using Storytelling to Build Emotional, Social and Academic Skills across the Primary Curriculum
Jennifer M. Fox Eades
ISBN 978 1 84310 304 2

Talking with Children and Young People about Death and Dying
2nd edition
Mary Turner
Illustrated by Bob Thomas
ISBN 978 1 84310 441 4

A Safe Place for Caleb
An Interactive Book for Kids, Teens and Adults with Issues of Attachment, Grief, Loss or Early Trauma
Kathleen A. Chara and Paul J. Chara, Jr.
Illustrated by J.M. Berns
ISBN 978 1 84310 799 6

Understanding Attachment and Attachment Disorders
Theory, Evidence and Practice
Vivien Prior and Danya Glaser
ISBN 978 1 84310 245 8
Child and Adolescent Mental Health series

Fostering Attachments
Supporting Children who are Fostered or Adopted
Kim S. Golding
ISBN 978 1 84310 614 2

Cool Connections with **Cognitive Behavioural Therapy**

Encouraging Self-esteem, Resilience and Well-being in Children and Young People Using CBT Approaches

Laurie Seiler

Jessica Kingsley Publishers
London and Philadelphia

All pages marked ✔ may be photocopied for use with this programme, but may not be reproduced for any other purpose without the permission of the publisher.

First published in 2008
by Jessica Kingsley Publishers
116 Pentonville Road
London N1 9JB, UK
and
400 Market Street, Suite 400
Philadelphia, PA 19106, USA

www.jkp.com

Library of Congress Cataloging in Publication Data

Seiler, Laurie.
  Cool connections with Cognitive Behavioural Therapy : encouraging self-esteem, resilience and well-being in children and young people using CBT approaches / Laurie Seiler.
      p. cm.
  ISBN 978-1-84310-618-0 (pb : alk. paper) 1. Cognitive therapy for children--Problems, exercises, etc. 2. Cognitive therapy for teenagers--Problems exercises, etc. I. Title.
  RJ505.C63S45 2008
  618.92'89142--dc22
                    2007033853

British Library Cataloguing in Publication Data
A CIP catalogue record for this book is available from the British Library

ISBN 978 1 84310 618 0

Printed and bound in Great Britain by
Printwise (Haverhill) Ltd, Suffolk

Contents

Preface

I would like to share a little information about myself, the Cool Connections Programme and its development. Having worked for a number of years within the caring professions, I qualified as a mental health nurse at Brunel University in 1997. Since then I have acquired a BSc (Hons) in specialist practice, a BA (Hons) in child and adolescent mental health studies, and a postgraduate diploma in cognitive behavioural therapy (CBT). I am now a fully accredited cognitive behavioural psychotherapist and registered with the British Association for Behavioural and Cognitive Psychotherapies (BABCP).

The Cool Connections Programme outlined in this workbook is a ten-session, early intervention group programme aimed at children aged 9–14. The programme is based on a cognitive behavioural approach and focuses on the prevention of anxiety and depression in children and young people. Included in this workbook is a facilitator's guide, which describes how to run the programme. Referral forms and home activity exercises are also included. The ten sessions are all illustrated and involve games, theory and numerous fun exercises.

My interest in creating a group programme for young people first developed following my work with children and families in Suffolk. Although there are several books with both interesting and creative ways of working with children, most focus either on older children or on young people with serious mental health difficulties, rather than early intervention. Of particular interest are the American group programme for working with anxious children, called Coping Cat, and the Australian programme, called Friends. The programme described in this workbook came about by combining the theory of CBT and building on existing ideas for group work exercises. Many of the exercises in the programme have been developed through trial and error and following evaluation by the many children who have taken part.

Acknowledgements

My thanks go to Dr Nicola Ridgeway who has supervised my CBT practice over the past few years and with whom I have shared many ideas for the programme. My good friend Ashley Barber has helped me with some of the IT ideas and computer technology. All members of the On Track team in Suffolk have supported me in putting the programme together, along with the many helpful comments made by the children who have taken part.

Group Facilitators' Guide to the Cool Connections Programme

Cool Connections is a ten-session early intervention programme aimed at children aged 9–14. The programme is based on a cognitive behavioural approach which aims to encourage self-esteem, social skills and well-being, and prevent anxiety and depression, in children and adolescents.

The group facilitators

The programme is written for those qualified to work with children, such as health care professionals, psychologists, teachers, social workers and youth counsellors. Unqualified staff can also facilitate the programme but they should spend time discussing and planning the group at least once every two weeks with a supervisor. The supervisor needs to be a qualified professional with experience of working with children and a good knowledge of confidentiality, safeguarding and child welfare issues. A background in the psychological therapies, or specific training in CBT, is a useful but not essential attribute for the group facilitators. So too is an experience of facilitating groups and an awareness of the implications of therapeutic work with children. Having said this, most professionals who facilitate the Cool Connections Programme will adapt the material to their own personal style and theoretical framework.

It is often helpful if the group is facilitated by two people. A qualified person might work, for example, with a teaching assistant based within the school. This helps provide the children with a supportive link person whom they see on a regular basis outside the group and encourages positive communication/relationships with teaching staff.

Aims of the programme

The aims of the programme include the following:

- Assist children and young people to develop life-skills to be able to cope effectively with difficult and/or anxiety-provoking situations.
- Normalize the emotional state of anxiety.
- Build emotional resilience and problem-solving abilities.
- Encourage peer learning and build peer support networks.
- Promote self-confidence in dealing with difficult, or anxiety-provoking, situations.
- Prevent anxiety and depression in children and young people.
- Mix with other children and have fun and positive experiences.

Evidence of effectiveness

The Cool Connections Programme has been successfully piloted within several schools in Suffolk over the past three years. It has also been run as an after-school group for children of different ages and as a family group programme where parents and children work together with other families. More than 150 children have taken part in this programme and several family groups have also been run. Feedback has been extremely positive from parents, teachers and participants. Measures of coping skills and self-esteem before and after the programme show all participants to date have reduced their levels of anxiety/depression by completing the programme. Individuals also report that the programme has been fun, helpful and informative.

Structure of the programme

The ten sessions include a mixture of fun games, educational material, therapeutic content and strategies. Participants will be involved in written exercises, discussion, role play, games, puppet work and art activities. They are encouraged to be creative in completing all the exercises and, where possible, interact, share experiences and work with each other in a way that helps normalize their experiences and increases social skills and confidence.

The first session aims to help children get to know each other and develop rapport with the facilitators. Sessions 2 to 5 help socialize the children to the cognitive model and increase awareness of thoughts, feelings, body signals and actions. Sessions 6 to 10 further educate the children and provide strategies to enable them to cope with the symptoms of anxiety and depression, for example by cognitive restructuring, problem-solving, goal-setting, breaking problems down into small steps (building a hierarchy), and using visualization techniques.

Each session in the programme follows the same framework as a cognitive behavioural therapy session:

- agenda setting
- Home activity review
- session content, including new material
- Home activity setting.

The Cool Connections Programme sessions generally move at quite a rapid pace and a lot of information and activities are covered in a short space of time. The exercises within each session are generally based on a single theme which is then presented in a range of different ways. It is not necessary, therefore, to complete every exercise in each session. Guidance as to which exercises are most important is provided in 'Agenda and tips for running the session', which is to be found at the start of each session. The essential exercises are shown in bold type. Depending on the facilitator's time frame and/or client group, it is fine to be flexible with regard to which of the other exercises are included or left out. Equally the facilitator may wish to incorporate his or her own material alongside that provided in each session. There are no hard and fast rules about this. It is fine to adapt the programme to suit individual styles, preferences and/or group needs.

In keeping with CBT protocol the group facilitator should aim to work in collaboration with the children or young people wherever possible. A scientific, evidence-based approach to problem solving is recommended.

Recruitment

Some of the groups we have run have contained children who have been specifically referred by parents or teaching staff. However, the best results have been generated when participants volunteer themselves for the programme. The way this works is that an assembly is held informing children in the school about the programme and inviting them to take part. Those interested are invited to complete a simple questionnaire (similar to the 'Feeling worried' exercise on pages 51–52 of Session 1), giving their name and reason for wishing to take part. Following consultation with school staff a group is then chosen. It is interesting to note that most children who volunteer themselves for the group programme are the same children many school staff identify as children 'in need'. Whilst in some clinical settings the volunteering approach may be impractical, encouraging children to volunteer themselves greatly enhances motivation, compliance and rapport building within the group.

In terms of group size, we have experimented with large groups of up to 14 children and smaller groups with as few as four children. From my experience single-sex groups with between six and eight children of a similar age work best with older children, though this may not be so crucial with younger children.

We have facilitated groups during school time, after school and had groups which included both parents and children together. In the latter case, the children and parents reported benefiting from the programme.

The setting

The environment for running the programme will depend on the facilities available. Teachers, for example, may prefer children to sit behind desks while health care workers may prefer a circle. Obviously, an environment conducive to learning is best achieved with a spacious, quiet room and a pleasant view. However, this is often not possible and facilitators will need to make the best of available resources. Very successful programmes can be run with limited resources and difficult working environments.

Support material

Each child in the group should have his or her own workbook. We have experimented by giving children complete ten-session workbooks at the start of the programme and also by providing children with A4 style ring binders where they add a session each week. With the complete workbook the ring binding gets damaged and/or children read ahead instead of focusing on the session in hand. The session-by-session approach works well and enables the facilitator to add or adapt material along the way. Some children like to add their home activity assignments to their folder as they are completed.

Time planning

The more time given to each session, the more the children will benefit. However, in many schools or organizations, time will be limited. For example, many of the sessions run by the author in schools have been restricted to one hour, which is usually the equivalent of one lesson in the school timetable. Although it is possible to run one session within this one-hour time frame, an hour and a half with a short break is preferable. This provides time to reflect on the previous week's home activity assignments, complete all the exercises/games in the programme, and discuss forthcoming home activity assignments. Additional material (videos, games, etc.) can also be included if required within this longer time frame. At the start of each session we have provided guidelines for 'short' sessions only one hour in duration and 'long' sessions lasting up to an hour and a half.

Homework

In line with cognitive behavioural theory, a home activity is given after each session and briefly reviewed with the children at the beginning of the following session. Two different home activities are provided for most sessions. The group facilitator can either choose one home activity or give the children both and let them choose which to complete. An enthusiastic group may choose to complete both. Unlike school homework, home activities are voluntary and the children complete them only if they choose to do so. However, it can be explained that they will get more from the programme if they do complete the extra work. In some groups we have offered a small reward for completing home activities to aid motivation, but this is not essential and is at the discretion of the facilitators.

The home activities are generally linked in some way to the content of that day's session. Most of the activities are intended to be fun and increase children's awareness of the relationship between their thoughts, feelings, body signals and actions (cognitive model). Research suggests that it is through this awareness that change can begin to take place. Children can write home activity feedback on the pages provided (see pages 34–35) at the facilitator's discretion.

Following each session group leaders are encouraged to meet and reflect upon each individual child and upon the session as a whole.

Difficulties in the group

Group facilitators, and organizations such as schools or child and adolescent mental health services, will have their own protocols for resolving difficulties that can present when working with groups of children. Facilitators will realize that some parts of the programme may require more skilled facilitation than others. For example, some exercises can be very upsetting for some children. If the distress is not addressed within the group this can lead to feelings of vulnerability and distrust.

The aim of Cool Connections is to help children cope with feelings of discomfort, and they are therefore encouraged to talk openly about their feelings. At times children may become quite upset and/or tearful in session. This can be viewed as a good thing as it suggests that the children are finding the group environment a safe place. However, there is little time allocated within each session to accommodate these feelings. Children's upset feelings need to be validated and empathy offered from within the group, at the same time acknowledging the possible impact on other group members. Children can choose whether to stay within the group for the session and/or discuss the issue with an appropriate adult on a one-to-one basis outside of the group. One of the facilitators can escort a child out of the group if required. From my experience children most frequently become upset during feedback at the beginning of the session. Exercises where children may require additional support include: 'Making cool connections' (page 69), 'Catching thoughts' (page 106), 'Your actions' (page 116), 'My cool connections' (page 120), 'My downward digger' (page 137), 'Red light thought challenge' (page 155), or 'Put safety first!' (page 179).

Confidentiality

In Session 1 the children are informed about confidentiality. At any point in the programme, if a child or parent raises issues regarding the safety of themselves or others (abuse, self-harm, drug taking, etc.), facilitators are advised to record the information given and follow the child safeguarding procedures within their organization. It is important children feel safe in the group or they are unlikely to share information. Children's confidentiality should be respected at all times throughout the programme. Any breach of confidentiality can be addressed openly with the group in the next session. Where appropriate this can be discussed without naming the individuals responsible.

Underlying principles of CBT

CBT involves development of a shared understanding or formulation of a client's problems. This understanding should inform both therapist and client regarding treatment. Unless each child were given a comprehensive cognitive behavioural assessment prior to undertaking the Cool Connections Programme, individual formulations would be difficult to achieve. Consequently, this programme is based on a cognitive behavioural 'approach' which should not be compared with CBT treatment with a trained therapist. However, the material in this programme, can be used both in conjunction with CBT treatment and as a useful resource for therapists working with children.

CBT encourages exploration of different ways of thinking, and therapists are encouraged to be non-judgemental in response to the children's thoughts and feelings. There are no right or wrong answers in this programme although some ways of thinking may be more useful in certain situations than others. The programme aims to increase children's awareness of thoughts, feelings, body signals and actions. It is suggested that through this awareness change can be initiated. Although it is in the nature of young children to think in polarized (black and white) ways, the programme is intended to encourage broader and more flexible thinking (looking for shades of grey) that promotes more acceptance and/or compassion towards the self and others and consequently a reduction in anxiety and/or stress levels.

The Cool Connections Programme and the National Curriculum

Within the UK the Cool Connections Programme has close links with the Government's Agenda for Change guidelines, 'Every Child Matters'. This approach involves the general well-being of all children and young people from birth to 19 years of age. The Government's aim is for every child, whatever their background or circumstances, to have the support they need to achieve the following five outcomes:

- be healthy
- stay safe
- enjoy and achieve
- make a positive contribution
- achieve economic well-being.

The Cool Connections Programme is closely linked with the National Curriculum, especially in relation to PSHE (Personal, Social and Health Education) guidelines at Key Stage 2 (7–11 years) and 3 (11–14 years). Links with Key Stage 2 targets are listed below:

- To talk and write about their opinions and explain their views on issues that affect themselves and society.
- To recognize their worth as individuals by identifying positive things about themselves and their achievements, seeing their mistakes, making amendments and setting personal goals.
- To face new challenges positively by collecting information, looking for help, making responsible choices and taking action.
- To see how their actions affect themselves and others, to care about other people's feelings and to try to see things from others' points of view.
- To learn where and how individuals, families and groups can get help and support.
- To reflect on spiritual, moral, social and cultural issues using imagination to understand other people's experiences.
- To resolve differences by looking at alternatives, making decisions and explaining choices.
- To understand what makes a healthy lifestyle, including the benefits of exercise and healthy eating, what affects mental health and how to make informed choices.
- To feel positive about themselves (for example, by producing personal diaries, profiles and portfolios of achievements, by having opportunities to show what they can do and how much responsibility they can take).

Links between the Cool Connections Programme and Key Stage 3 targets, in addition to the above, also include:

- To be able to recognize how others see them and be able to give and receive constructive feedback and praise.
- To understand how to keep healthy.
- To see that good relationships and an appropriate balance between work, leisure and exercise can promote physical and mental health.

- To understand how to empathize with people different from themselves.
- To communicate confidently with peers and adults.

Importance of early intervention and prevention programmes

The importance of early intervention programmes is accentuated by research that suggests children who suffer from high anxiety are more likely to become anxious adults (Mattison 1992). Early anxiety intervention programmes have been shown to reduce the number of children and young people developing anxiety disorders. Furthermore, such programmes are cost-effective, in a group-based approach reducing the cost of future professional services, as well as targeting a number of individuals simultaneously over a short period of time. In short, effective early intervention programmes represent a significant opportunity to prevent a great deal of suffering for individuals and their families.

Reference

Mattison, R.E. (1992) 'Anxiety Disorders.' In S.R. Hooper, G.W. Hynd and R.E. Mattison (eds) *Child Psychopathology: Diagnostic Criteria and Clinical Assessment.* Hillsdale, NJ: Lawrence Erlbaum Associates.

Cognitive Behavioural Therapy

The Cool Connections Programme is rooted in the theory of cognitive behavioural therapy (CBT). In this section I give a brief summary of the theory and principles of the approach. If a facilitator is keen to find out more about the approach I have included a number of references for further reading.

Cognitive behavioural therapy is a relatively new method of psychotherapy that emerged in the 1950s and is considered to have evolved from the ideas of Pavlov and Skinner (Salkovskis 1996). The approach is generally associated with the work of Albert Ellis and Aaron Beck that dates back to the early 1970s. The model for CBT arose from Beck's cognitive therapy for depression in the 1960s when he proposed that depressed people are prone to thinking in a distorted way and that they typically have a negative view of themselves, the world and other people (Tarrier 2006). In the 1980s the cognitive therapists joined forces with behavioural therapists to help challenge people's inaccurate beliefs. The two therapies merged to form the backbone of the CBT approach.

The therapy has more recently been seen as a short-term structured approach that involves collaboration between the individual with the problem and the therapist to achieve certain goals. Unlike psychoanalytical psychotherapy, CBT is an evidence-based approach which aims to resolve current problems rather than drawing upon assumptions made by the therapist commonly relating to past (unresolved) conflicts. CBT focuses on what the problem is now, what is maintaining it and what can be done to alleviate it (Persons 1989). In CBT the therapist is considered to work with individuals to help them identify thoughts, feelings and behaviours associated with their problems. Clients are also encouraged to explore different ways of thinking and to consider alternative interpretations of their beliefs. It is further suggested that when clients have developed these skills they can also learn new behaviours and problem-solving strategies with which to reinterpret their thoughts, feelings and behaviours in more rational ways.

There is growing interest in the use of CBT with children and young people. This interest has been encouraged by a number of reviews which conclude that CBT is a promising and effective intervention for the treatment of child psychological problems (Rapee *et al.* 2000). CBT in this age group is seen as an intervention that aims to promote emotional and behavioural change by teaching children to change their thoughts and thought processes in an overt, active and problem-solving manner. In Kendall and Mac-Donald's (1993) conceptualization of the model they suggest children may be helped to identify distorted processing and be guided towards modifying their distorted thinking. Friedberg and McClure (2002) echo this, stating that anxieties, fears and worries are commonplace childhood occurrences. They report that, according to the cognitive model, five spheres of functioning change when children are anxious: physiological, mood, behavioural, cognitive and interpersonal. It has been suggested that treatment for childhood anxieties generally focuses on quietening down distressing symptoms by providing increased coping skills (Friedberg and McClure 2002):

> CBT is the current 'wonder' treatment and in guidelines published by the National Institute for Clinical Excellence (NICE), CBT has been recommended as the treatment of choice for a number of conditions ranging from post-traumatic stress disorder to depression. At this point in time CBT has established itself as the therapy for children most strongly backed by scientific evidence although the evidence base is still quite limited. (Stallard 2007)

Although the literature on the treatment of children and adolescents with CBT is far less extensive than that for adults, a number of studies – mostly conducted in the last four to five years – have confirmed the short-term efficacy and safety of treatments for anxiety and depression in young people. A study supported by the National Alliance on Mental Illness (NAMI 2007) comparing different types of psychotherapy for major depression in children found that CBT led to remission in nearly 65 per cent of cases, a higher rate than that following either supportive therapy or family therapy. CBT also resulted in a more rapid treatment response. Results are higher in relation to children with anxiety. Children with anxiety are reported to have approximately a 70 to 80 per cent response rate with CBT, and the gains are maintained over time.

Until recently it has been suggested that young children are unlikely to understand cognitive concepts and therefore will not benefit from CBT. Consequently, play or systematic family therapy have been considered more appropriate treatments. However, in recent years there has been increasing evidence that CBT may be effective with both children and adolescents. With parental support, children as young as two or three can learn how to use non-anxious self-talk (using puppets or dolls as models) and desensitization through gradual exposure.

Stallard (2002) proposes that CBT approaches with young people need to be modified to coincide with the individual's developmental stage and cognitive abilities. It is suggested that it is the way the CBT material is presented that needs to change as opposed to the approach being inappropriate. He notes that you would not expect to achieve positive outcomes with children when applying unadapted adult tools.

The CBT approach is considered to help children challenge their thoughts and understanding of situations, rather than accepting their thoughts as the truth. CBT encourages children to generate more realistic versions of situations and their ability to cope with them. Ready with a new mindset, children then gradually face difficult or fearful situations, breaking the challenges down into small, manageable steps. Over time, children are able to tap more quickly into non-anxious interpretations of situations, and in some cases understand that avoidance of feared situations can help maintain their difficulties.

With an increasing number of studies in recent years providing empirical evidence of the effectiveness of CBT with children, both on an individual basis and in groups, there is a strong case for using CBT to achieve the kinds of long-term improvements in children and young people described in this summary. Stallard reflects this, stating: 'Effectiveness needs to be substantiated and there is a national need to improve the availability and practice of CBT with children and young people' (Stallard 2007).

References

Friedberg, R.D. and McClure, J.M. (2002) *Clinical Practice of Cognitive Therapy with Children and Adolescents: The Nuts and Bolts.* New York: Guilford Press.

Kendall, P.C. and MacDonald, J.P. (1993) 'Cognition in the Psychopathology of Youth and Implications for Treatment.' In K.S. Dobson and P.C. Kendall (eds), *Psychopathology and Cognition* (pp.387-427). California: Academic Press.

NAMI (2007) *Helpline Facts Sheet: Children and Adolescent OCD.* Accessed on 11/01/08 at www.nami.org/helpline/ocd.htm.

Persons, J.B. (1989) *Cognitive Therapy in Practice: A Case Formulation Approach.* New York: W.W. Norton & Company.

Rapee, R.M., Wignall, A., Hudson, J.L and Schniering, C.A. (2000) *Treating Anxious Children and Adolescents: An Evidence-Based Approach.* Oakland, CA: New Harbinger Publications.

Salkovskis, P.M. (1996) *Frontiers of Cognitive Therapy.* New York: Guilford Press.

Stallard, P. (2002) *Think Good Feel Good: A Cognitive Behaviour Therapy Workbook for Children.* Chichester: John Wiley & Sons, Ltd.

Stallard, P. (2007) 'Expert's Concerns about Child Mental Health Services.' Accessed on 11/01/08 at www.bath.ac.uk/news/2007/4/11/paulstallardlecture.html.

Tarrier, N. (ed.) (2006) *Case Formulation in Cognitive Behaviour Therapy: The Treatment of Challenging and Complex Cases.* Oxford: Oxford University Press.

Useful Links and References

The programme acknowledges the ideas and inspiration of others who have gone before, including the following:

Alexander, J. (2003) *Bullies, Bigmouths and So-called Friends.* London: Hodder Children's Books.

British Association for Behavioural and Cognitive Psychotherapies: www.BABCP.com

Chansky, T.E. (2004) *Freeing Your Child from Anxiety: Powerful, Practical Solutions to Overcome Your Child's Fears, Worries, and Phobias.* New York: Broadway Books.

Friedberg, R.D. (2001) *Therapeutic Exercises for Children Workbook: Guided Self-Discovery Using Cognitive-Behavioral Techniques.* Sarasota, FL: Professional Resource Exchange, Inc.

Friends (an Australian programme designed for the prevention of anxiety and depression in children and youths): www.friendsinfo.net

Huebner, D. (2005) *What to Do When You Worry Too Much: A Kid's Guide to Overcoming Anxiety.* Washington, DC: Magination Press.

Kendall, P.C. and Hedtke, K.A (2006) *The Coping Cat Workbook, 2nd Edition.* Ardmore, PA: Workbook Publishing, Inc.

Rapee, R.M., Spence, S.H., Cobham, V. and Wignall, A. (2000) *Helping Your Anxious Child: A Step-by-Step Guide for Parents.* Oakland, CA: New Harbinger Publications .

Rapee, R.M., Wignall, A., Hudson, J.L and Schniering, C.A. (2000) *Treating Anxious Children and Adolescents: An Evidence-Based Approach.* Oakland, CA: New Harbinger Publications.

Stallard, P. (2002) *Think Good Feel Good: A Cognitive Behaviour Therapy Workbook for Children.* Chichester: John Wiley & Sons, Ltd.

Stark, K. and Kendall, P.C (1996) *Treating Depressed Children: Therapist Manual for "Taking Action".* Ardmore, PA: Workbook Publishing, Inc.

PRE-GROUP MATERIAL

Pre-group Material Contents

Individual recording sheet

Facilitators are encouraged to record information following sessions. They may find this a useful format for recording information about individuals.

Assessment tool: What RU like?

For those facilitators able to offer a one-to-one session to children before the programme begins. This tool aims to provide some background information and help build rapport between children and the facilitators before the group begins.

Cool Connections Programme self-referral form

Useful form that children can complete themselves to take part in the programme (following a school assembly for example).

Home activity feedback

Some children or facilitators may find it useful to record what individual children have learned from their home activities each week.

Individual recording sheet

Name: **Group facilitator(s):**

Date / session number	Comments

Date / session number	Comments

Date / session number	Comments

Date / session number	Comments

Date / session number	Comments

Date / session number	Comments

Date / session number	Comments

Date / session number	Comments

Date / session number	Comments

Date / session number	Comments

Assessment tool: What RU like?

My favourite things are...	
My friends say I am...	
My mum is...	
My dad is...	
My school is...	
I feel angry about...	
The things I'm sad about are...	
The things I'm frightened of are...	
I don't like...	
My secret is...	
If I had a magic wand I would...	
If I could ask one question without upsetting anyone I would ask...	

Adapted from Herbert, M. (1991) *Clinical Child Psychology: Social Learning, Development and Behaviour.* Chichester: Wiley.

Cool Connections Programme self-referral form

We are running a group to help children cope with their feelings. The group will involve some fun games, acting, stories, art work and learning more about feelings. If you want to join the group complete the information below.

What is your name?

How often do you worry or feel sad about things? Tick the box which best describes you.

Never	Sometimes	Every day

Where do you feel most sad or worried? Tick the box which best describes you.

Never	Sometimes	Every day

Why do you think you should be included in the Cool Connections Programme?

Home activity feedback

What did you learn or notice from your homework this week?

1

2

3

4

5

6

7

8

9

10

SESSIONS

Session 1: Getting to Know Each Other

Aims and objectives

- Enable group members to get to know each other.
- Agree some group rules.
- Begin learning about feelings and make some goals.
- Begin sharing feelings with other members of the group.
- Have fun.

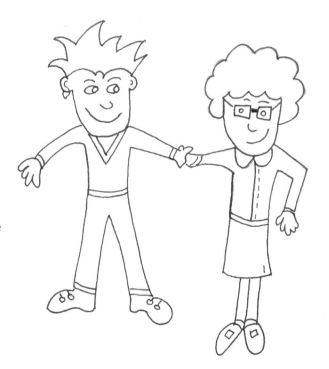

Materials

Chairs, pencils.

Agenda and tips for running the session

Exercises in bold in the left-hand column should be included in both long and short sessions. Many fun activities/games are included as optional. Despite sometimes being short of time it is important not to cut all the 'fun' out of the programme or you will lose the children's enthusiasm.

Short session

EXERCISE	COMMENTS
Welcome children	Share agenda for session with group.
Meet the gang	There are four characters who feature throughout the programme: Jack, Harry, Lauren and Katie. This exercise introduces the characters to the group.
All change game	This game can be adapted to suit the group. The general aim is to help children relax and get to know each other.
Confidentiality	Important to share this for professional reasons and to develop trust within the group.
Group rules	Give the children a list of the rules (see page 47 or make up your own). The group members can sign and return for the next session. This is only a guide. Group facilitators may choose to alter or change the rules at their discretion.
Who am I?	Having completed this exercise ask children to feed back two bits of information about themselves of their choice. This might include only their name.
Feeling worried	Read the paragraph at the top of the first page and take one or two examples from the children without completing the boxes.
Rate yourself	Children frequently find this difficult. It is better if they can be specific about areas in their life that they hope taking part in the group will help with. Where children have difficulty coming up with things for themselves or identifying their own personal problems they can be asked questions such as: 'If a friend had the chance to be involved in this programme what do you think it would help him with?' At this stage in the programme children can be given the choice whether they share information with the rest of the group or not.

'Flipping your lid'

Some children are very self-conscious about acting (page 54), especially in the first session. This can be overcome by encouraging children to draw a picture or just talk about a scenario with a friend without acting. This self-consciousness can provide information about some children's anxiety and it can be very helpful to encourage them to work through this. Our experience is that the children's confidence grows as the programme progresses.

Home Activity 1a:
My family

Children can complete this in any way they choose (stick men are fine). This activity helps children get to know one another better. It also provides facilitators with more information about an individual's support network. Much can be gained from close observation of the children's drawings, for example who they include or miss out from pictures, and who is close to whom – also facial characteristics. It is important to check out with the children observations taken from drawings rather than jumping to conclusions. Quality of drawings is unimportant but may help facilitators identify personality traits: perfectionism, etc.

Home Activity 1b:
Hopes and dreams

This activity helps children to be specific about their difficulties and their goals and helps them generate some solutions of their own. There is much research suggesting that the clearer you can imagine your dreams for the future the closer you become to making them reality. The drawings only have to mean something to the children. The exercise encourages children to visualize their difficulties and how they could be resolved. It could be used in place of the rating scales on pages 53 and 200, compared with pictures drawn at the end of the programme.

Long session

As above but more time can be spent on warm-up games. Group rules can be discussed in session and created by the children. The 'Feeling worried' exercise can be completed in full.

Notes

The most important aspect of this session is to give the children a positive experience and for them to begin to get to know one another. This helps in developing trust and in normalizing the children's feelings. It can be very therapeutic to see that other children have worries/problems too. There are a lot of different activities in this first session. You may choose to change the games or activities to suit your time frame.

Meet the gang

Meet the following four characters below. They will be helping you by offering pictures and examples as you work through the Cool Connections Programme. From the pictures and thought bubbles shown in the programme you may assume the following about each of the characters.

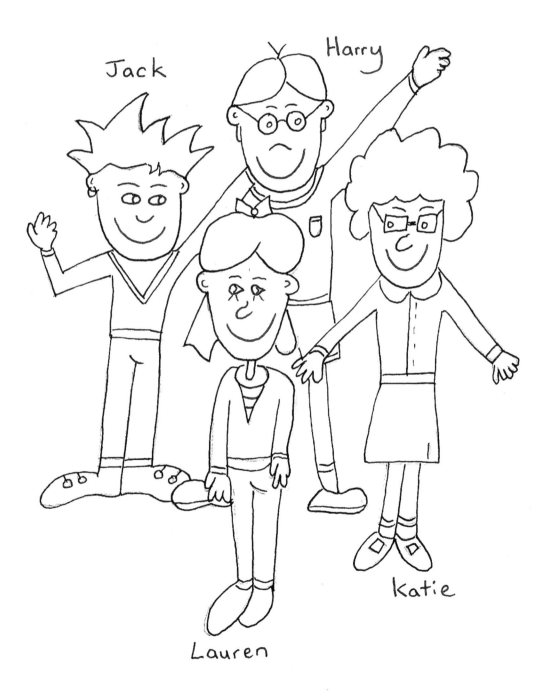

Jack: Fun to be with and good at sports. Especially likes football and often comes up with good ideas. Sometimes at school he thinks he is stupid and worries about making mistakes. Jack's parents often argue and shout at him at home. This often makes him feel angry inside. Jack is very scared of spiders. He can also be mean to Katie at times.

Harry: Harry really likes snooker, climbing and computers. He is also good at building things. Harry is very fond of Lauren and sometimes dreams of being a superhero. He has poor eyesight which upsets him at times and he is very frightened of snakes and worries about his health. He likes climbing and sometimes talks about other children behind their backs. Harry does not get on well with his teacher at school.

Katie: Likes to relax in the sunshine and likes the company of Jack. She tends to opt out of things and does not like sports. Katie can be bossy towards other children and thinks of herself as both fat and ugly. Sometimes when she is with other people she tries to hide her unhappy feelings by wearing a 'happy' mask. Katie can sometimes be bossy towards other children and has a quick temper when things don't go her way.

Lauren: Popular with other children and enjoys lots of activities such as diving, tennis and dancing. She is also good at science subjects at school. Despite being popular Lauren often worries about what other people think of her and tries to please others. However, she has been known to be cruel to animals. Lauren's family are very important to her and she worries about being away from them. Although she can be very supportive of others she can be a gossip with her friends.

All change game

'All change' is an easy game to play. It is a fun way of getting to know other group members and making cool connections with each other. To play the game group members sit in a circle facing each other on their chairs. The group facilitator shouts 'all change' and everyone swaps seats. After a few turns one chair is taken away. When everyone has changed chairs the person left in the middle tells the group something about themselves then shouts 'all change'. The game can be repeated as many times as you like. This game helps you to get to know each other and to learn how people are different.

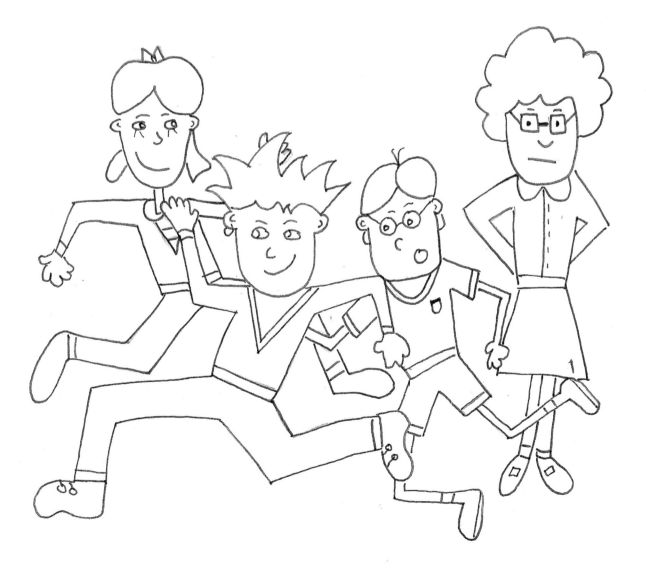

Confidentiality

'Confidentiality' means that what we talk about in the group is special to the group and we won't tell anyone outside the group about it without asking the group first.

It's OK for you to talk to your own family and friends about what *you* do and say in the group if you want to, but remember, what *others* say is private.

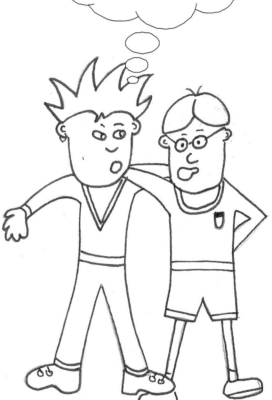

Have you heard what Lauren said in the group?

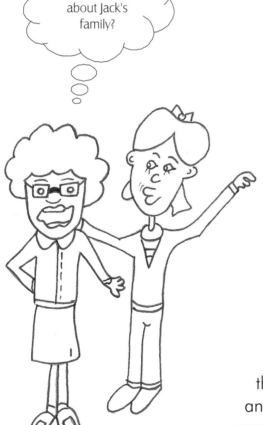

Did you hear about Jack's family?

If you tell the group facilitators anything that makes them think that you are not safe outside the group or that you are in danger they will have to talk to someone outside the group who can help protect you. But they will try to tell you what they are doing and why. The most important thing is that you are *safe*.

Group rules

Respect each other

It is important that we each try to respect other children in the group and the group facilitators. This involves supporting and listening to each other and taking turns to speak.

Timekeeping

It makes it difficult if you are not on time for the group to start. While it is the responsibility of the group facilitators to ensure groups are organized to start and finish on time, it is your responsibility not to be late.

Personal choice

It is your choice to be in the group. By making this choice you can decide to leave at any time. However, for safety reasons it is important that you let the group facilitators know of your whereabouts at all times. If you are disrupting the group your actions will suggest that you no longer wish to take part and you will be given the choice to either stay and stop disrupting the session or leave the group. If you choose to leave on more than one occasion you may be asked to leave the group altogether.

Commitment

It is important that if you are to get something out of this group then you are prepared to put something in of yourself. We hope to encourage all of the group to take part in all the activities. However, we will not make anyone do anything. By making the commitment to become part of the group you also commit to doing the home activity work and taking part in all group activities, not just the ones you like.

I agree to keep to the group rules and to stick to the confidentiality agreement

Signature: _

Who am I?

Complete the following sentences about yourself.

My name is:

The people in my family are:

I like to:

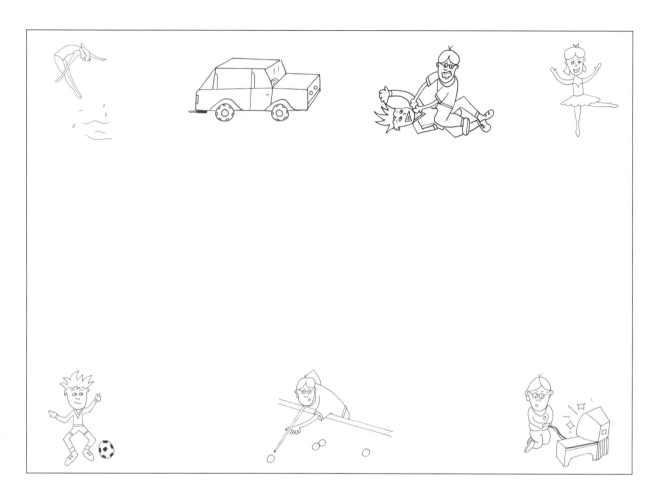

The worst thing in my life is:

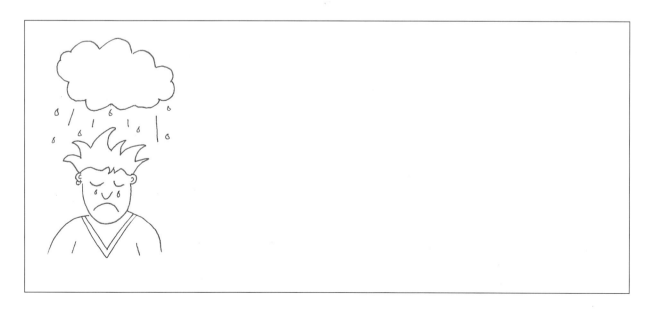

Nice things my friends say about me are:

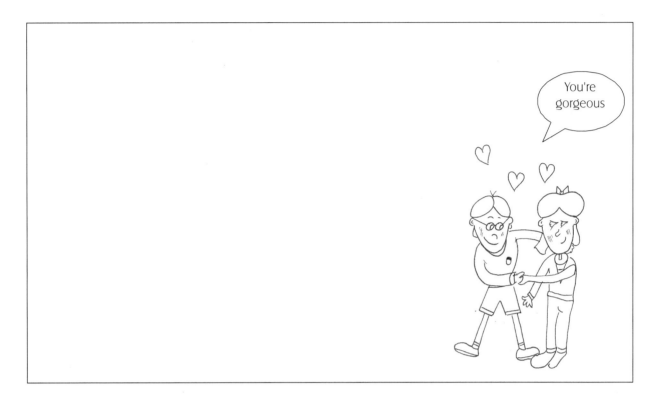

One thing I would like to change about myself is:

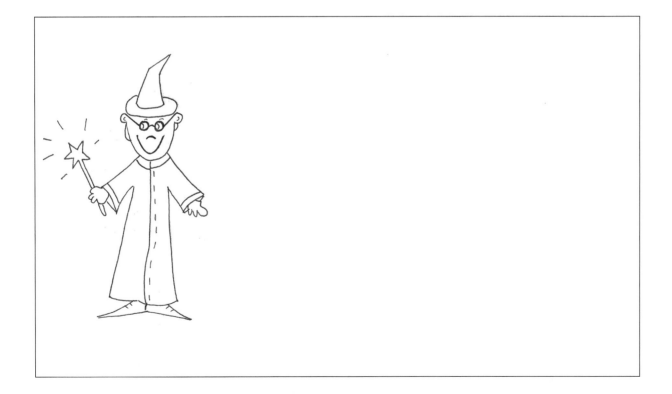

Feeling worried

Everyone has feelings and gets worried sometimes no matter how old or young they are. People get scared about different things too. Some children are scared of animals like snakes or bears while others worry about things such as the dark or heights. Sometimes children worry about making new friends, going to parties, doing school work or being away from their mums, dads or home. Whatever it is that makes each of us feel worried, being afraid is a feeling everyone has sometimes.

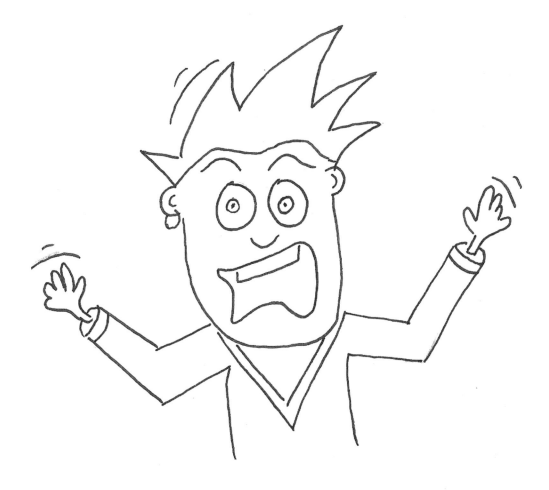

Below are some of the things lots of children worry about. Please tick the boxes which best describe your worries. If there are any things you worry about that are not on the list write them in the empty spaces at the bottom.

Spiders	Hospitals	Going to school	Snakes	The dark
Arguments at home	Speaking out in class	Keeping my family safe	Germs and dirt	Being told off
Eating in front of other kids	Being sick	Using the telephone	Being bullied	Making mistakes
Scary thoughts I can't get rid of	Being away from mum and dad	Not having many friends	Feeling I have to do things over and over again	Being fat and ugly
Secrets I can't talk about to do with home or school	What other kids think about me	Getting a serious illness like cancer or AIDS	What happens when I die	Being attacked

Rate yourself

Mark a cross on the number you currently feel most represents your life and how you are coping at the moment both in and out of school.

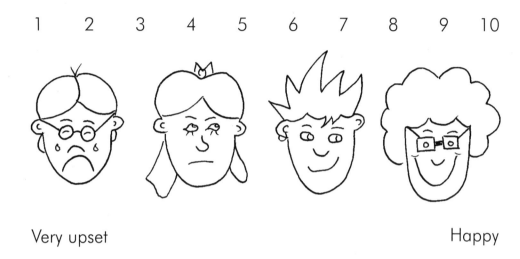

| 1 | 2 | 3 | 4 | 5 | 6 | 7 | 8 | 9 | 10 |

Very upset   Happy

List three things below which you feel most upset about in your life at the moment. Put a cross on the number which best represents how you feel.

Example: _ _ _ _ _ _ _ _ _ _ _ _ I have not got many friends _ _ _ _ _ _ _ _ _ _ _ _ _

1   2̶   3   4   5   6   7   8   9   10
Very upset   Happy

1. _

1   2   3   4   5   6   7   8   9   10
Very upset   Happy

2. _

1   2   3   4   5   6   7   8   9   10
Very upset   Happy

3. _

1   2   3   4   5   6   7   8   9   10
Very upset   Happy

'Flipping your lid'

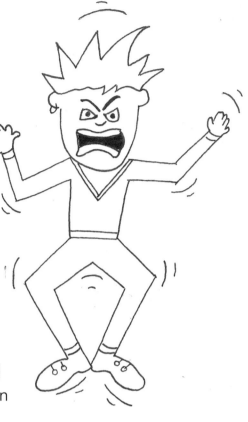

It happens all the time. People 'flip their lids' when they get worried, upset, or lose their cool. This is often caused by something called stress.

Everyone becomes stressed from time to time. It can affect doctors, teachers, dancers, sportsmen, drivers, and shop workers too. Mothers and fathers can become stressed when they can't pay the bills, when they have too much work to do, or when there are long queues on the roads or in the supermarkets. Children also can become stressed when they can't understand their school work, when other children pick on them, or when adults don't listen to them.

The trouble with stress is that it often gets passed on from one person to another. For example, if business is poor, the boss gets upset with an employee. During lunch, the employee is rude to a waitress. The waitress goes home that night and scolds her children. Finally the children yell at the cat. But what is the poor cat supposed to do?

People often behave differently when they are under stress. People can start to shout or act like wild animals. Some people growl and roar like tigers; others go crazy like wild monkeys. Some people even lose control and charge like rhinoceroses breaking up everything in sight. Still others become quiet and hide away like a tortoise in its shell. Some people cry real crocodile tears while others refuse to face the problem and bury their heads in the sand like ostriches.

In the Cool Connections Programme we are going to look at some cool ways to cope with those bottled-up feelings which cause stress and can cause people to 'flip their lids'. These feelings include fear, anger, sadness and guilt.

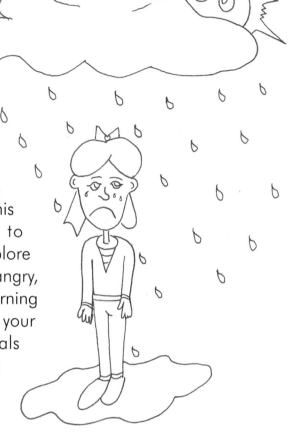

You will learn to become more aware of your thoughts, feelings, body signals and actions. With this information you can learn to recognize your feelings and explore new ways to cope when you feel angry, worried, down or stressed. By learning the 'cool connections' between your thoughts, feelings, body signals and actions you will become less likely to 'flip your lid' and more likely to 'stay cool'!

Think of a time when you have felt unhappy and stressed. With a friend act out the scene and show it to the group.

Give a brief description of the scene you acted within this box:

Home Activity 1a: My family

Draw a picture of your family. Include yourself in the picture.

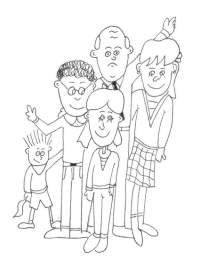

Home Activity 1b: Hopes and dreams

On the lines below list two things you hope the group will help you with:

1. _

   _

2. _

   _

In the box below draw one of your main worries or problems:

BOX 1

In the box below draw what your worry or problem would look like 'all better'.

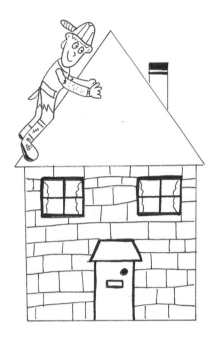

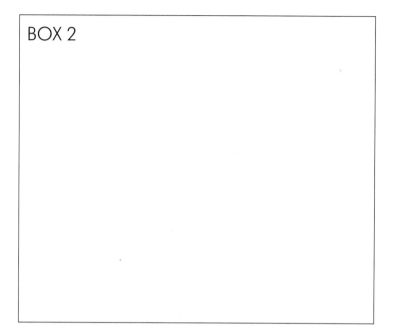

BOX 2

In the box below draw a way you could get from Box 1 (your problem) to Box 2 (your 'all better').

BOX 3

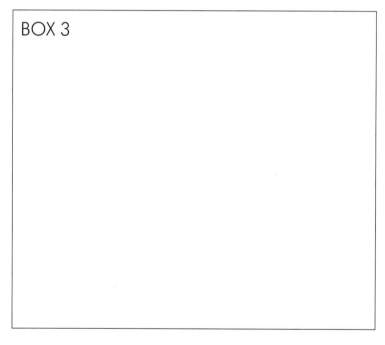

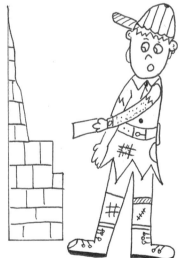

Session 2: Identify Different Feelings

Aims and objectives

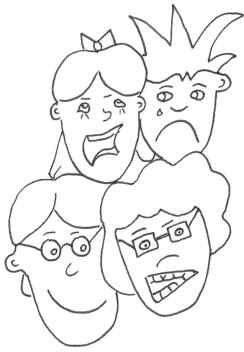

- Learn about different feelings.
- Notice how others may be feeling by looking at their faces and body language.
- Learn how feelings change all the time throughout each day.
- Begin seeing a connection between the way we feel and what we think.

Materials

Pencils, drawing paper, feelings dice (cube or square box with different feelings – happy, sad, worried, etc. – stuck to each side).

Agenda and tips for running the session

Exercises in bold in the left-hand column should be included in both long and short sessions. Many fun activities/games are included as optional. Despite sometimes being short of time it is important not to cut all the 'fun' out of the programme or you will lose the children's enthusiasm.

Short session

EXERCISE	COMMENTS
Feedback	Welcome children and share agenda for session with the group. Gain brief feedback from group members about their week. This feedback needs to be very brief or it can quickly consume the majority of the session. One piece of information from each child is recommended. If children provide upsetting or concerning feedback at this time empathy should be given, and one-to-one time to discuss the issue in detail is recommended following the session.
Review home activities from Session 1	Children can briefly show their drawings from Home Activities 1a and 1b. Group facilitators collect home activities to explore in more detail after the session and return the following week or at the end of the programme.
Feelings frenzy	Fun game to help children identify different feelings. A feelings dice is required.
What 'r' feelings?	Some children enjoy reading and can be made to feel more involved. However, this can slow the session down.
Name that feeling	Children are invited to share with the group and compare their answers with other group members.
Different feelings	This exercise aims to show children that people can have different feelings in the same situation. Three or four children from the group are asked to share the feelings they have identified. Group facilitators encourage the children to identify connections between their feelings and actions. For example, Jack circled that he felt scared when he saw the spider and that he would scream. Alternatively, Lauren felt excited and would pick the spider up.

Act how you feel game	As in Session 1, some children may feel self-conscious and the activity can be adapted if necessary. For example, children may act with a partner but not in front of the group.
Making cool connections	In this exercise the children are further encouraged to make connections between how they feel and what they do. There may only be time for the children to complete one example and to share with the group if they wish. Children are encouraged to draw 'stick people' rather than complex figures to save time.
Home Activity 2a: How do you feel?	This activity continues to help children make connections between their feelings and actions. It also creates an awareness of problem areas in their lives and begins to provide a range of words to describe their feelings.
Home Activity 2b: Activity and feelings record	This type of activity record is frequently seen in the CBT literature. It can have many functions with regard to therapy. For the purpose of this programme the activity record is aimed at increasing awareness of activities and the effect that these activities have on children's mood/actions. Depressed or anxious children often think that they feel this way all the time. Recording feelings in this way can be a useful way of testing this out. Children can be encouraged to do more of the activities they notice make them feel good and perhaps use problem-solving techniques (see Session 8) to cope better with activities which make them feel low or anxious.

Long session

More time can be spent over feedback and in the 'Act how you feel game'. Children can also be shown video/DVD clips or pictures and asked to guess the feelings of different characters. Children can be asked to discuss the characters' body language and how this can provide us with visual information about how people are feeling. Role plays are also a useful way both to portray feelings and to gain insight into the feelings of others.

Notes

All the children can be encouraged to feed back on every exercise. The session could also include a video/DVD or picture cards showing different feelings. These could be used as an alternative to the 'Feelings frenzy' activity. Children have to identify different feelings and suggest what this tells them from what they can hear/see that the person in the picture is experiencing.

Feelings frenzy

- All children sit in a circle facing each other.
- One child volunteers to start in the middle. He/she throws the feelings dice. Depending what feeling the dice lands on he/she must name a time, place or situation which goes with that feeling. For example: scared = when I saw a spider; excited = going to the fairground, etc.
- After naming a place or situation the child in the centre of the circle shouts 'feelings frenzy'.
- Any children who would share that feeling in the given situation change seats. Any one who would not share the feeling stands on their chair.
- The person left without a chair is next to throw the feelings dice.

Example: Lauren is in the middle of the circle. She throws the feelings dice which lands on a happy face. She informs the group that she is happy when she is at home. Jack does not feel happy at home so he stands on his chair. Harry and Katie do feel happy at home so they rush to change places. Lauren beats Harry to Katie's seat, leaving Harry in the middle to start the game again.

What 'r' feelings?

We all experience different feelings. They are what we feel inside about people, places or situations, e.g. happy, sad, angry or afraid. Becoming able to identify and name different feelings is the first important step to making cool connections about yourself and other people. Share an example of a feeling with the rest of the group. Notice how many different feelings there are.

Feelings can change from minute to minute and day to day depending on your situation. For example, if you are running in a race you may feel happy or excited, yet if by accident you fall over and hurt yourself your feelings may change and you become upset or angry.

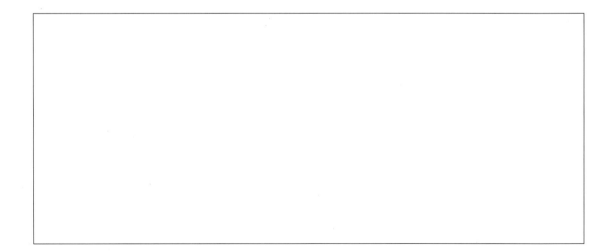

In the box below describe a time when you noticed your feelings change from one feeling to another very suddenly.

Some people think that feelings are good or bad but that is not true. They are just feelings, and feelings are neither good nor bad. It is OK to feel angry, upset or worried. It is also OK to tell others how you feel but it is not OK to hurt other people or break things. Sometimes people can have more than one different type of feeling at the same time.

For example:

- Jack loved his younger sister because she was good fun but he also hated her for breaking his favourite game.

- Lauren felt really excited about going on a fairground ride but she also felt a bit nervous too.

- The man was happy and sad about a pet who died (happy his pet was no longer in pain but sad that his pet is no longer with him).

Can you share with the group a time that you had more than one feeling at the same time?

Name that feeling

You can sometimes tell how other people are feeling by looking at their faces. From the list at the bottom of the page make cool connections by linking the face with the feeling. There are no right or wrong answers. It's up to you.

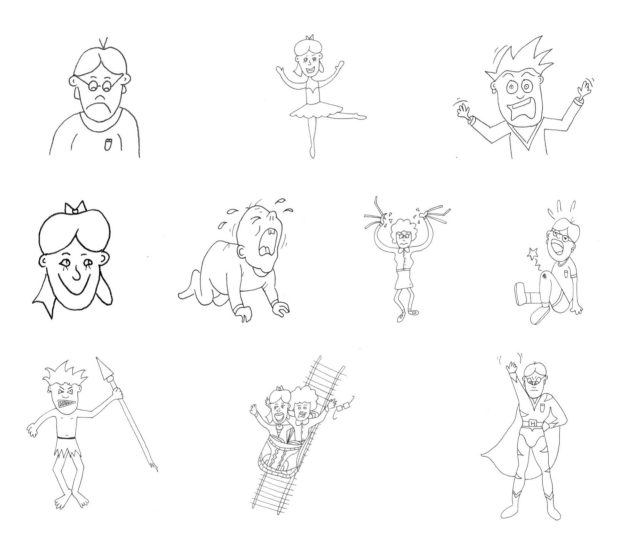

Happy	Excited	Frustrated	Upset	Tearful
Angry	Scared	Sad	Joyful	Powerful

Different feelings

Before you came to this group today how were you feeling?

Excited	Nervous	Bored	Frustrated
Angry	Upset	Apprehensive	Disappointed
Overjoyed	Sad	Terrified	Relaxed

How would you feel if you saw a giant spider climbing up your chair?

Excited	Nervous	Bored	Frustrated
Angry	Upset	Apprehensive	Disappointed
Overjoyed	Sad	Terrified	Relaxed

How would you feel if a kind teacher gave you all some liquorice sweets?

Excited	Nervous	Bored	Frustrated
Angry	Upset	Apprehensive	Disappointed
Overjoyed	Sad	Terrified	Relaxed

Feed back your answers to the rest of the group.

What did you notice?

Did other children answer the same as you?

What does this say about feelings?

Act how you feel game

- Find a partner from within the group.
- Act or draw a situation where someone has a strong feeling. This can be real or made up (e.g. being bullied = anger; a shark attack = fear).
- Act or draw your scene and let the other group members guess what is happening. The other group members can try and identify which feelings you are demonstrating.

Briefly describe the scene you drew or acted in the box below. Which feelings were you demonstrating?

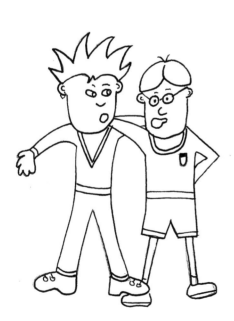

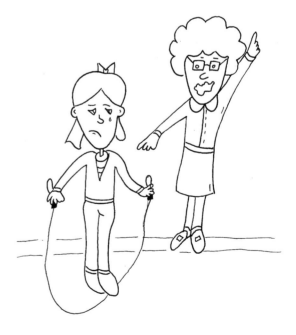

Making cool connections

Write something which makes you feel *happy*.

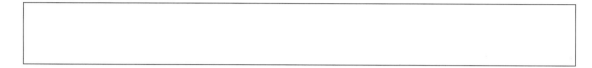

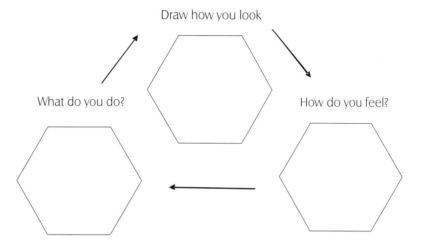

Write something which makes you feel *worried or scared*.

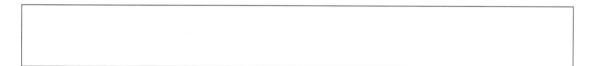

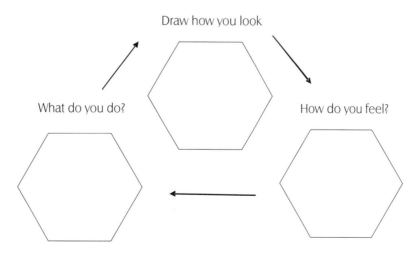

Write something which makes you feel *angry or cross*.

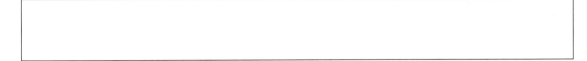

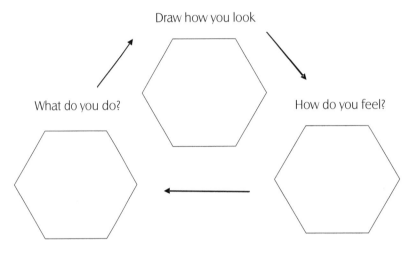

Draw how you look

What do you do?

How do you feel?

Write something which makes you feel *sad or down*.

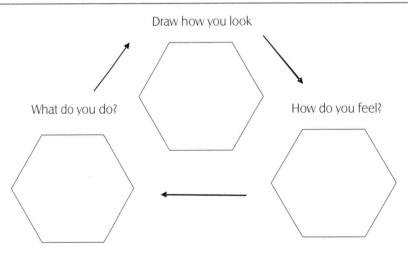

Draw how you look

What do you do?

How do you feel?

Home Activity 2a: How do you feel?

Link the feelings with the situations below:

At school	In bed at night	With my friends
While out in the town	Sharing my feelings	With my mum or dad

Happy	Sad	Bored
Relaxed	Angry	Frightened
Frustrated	Upset	Excited
Lonely	Guilty	Confused

Home Activity 2b: Activity and feelings record

- Write the important things you have done this week in the boxes below (e.g. watching TV, maths, football, etc.).

- Write your feelings next to the activities, e.g. happy, sad, worried, etc.

- Give your feeling a score out of 10 depending on the strength of feeling: 1 = not much, 10 = very strong.

- If you find room you could also draw what your face looked like at the time.

	MONDAY	TUESDAY	WEDNESDAY	THURSDAY	FRIDAY	SATURDAY	SUNDAY
MORNING							
LUNCH							
AFTERNOON							
EVENING							

SESSION 3: Body Signals and Biology

Aims and objectives

- Enable the group to become aware of the physical changes in their bodies.
- Learn the connection between body signals and the way we think, feel and behave.

Materials

Chairs, pencils.

Agenda and tips for running the session

Exercises in bold in the left-hand column should be included in both long and short sessions. Other exercises are optional and can be included in groups where there is more time. Many fun activities/games are included as optional. Despite sometimes being short of time it is important not to cut all the 'fun' out of the programme or you will lose the children's enthusiasm.

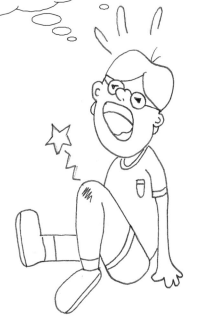

Short session

EXERCISE	COMMENTS
Feedback	Welcome the children and share agenda for session with group. Obtain brief feedback from children's week.
Review home activity	Children can briefly show their work, etc. Questions may be asked about the previous week's homework. Facilitators collect home activities to explore in more detail after the session and return the following week or at the end of the programme.
Tense and floppy game	The aim is to increase children's awareness of the physical changes in their bodies and notice the difference between tense and floppy muscles. This can also be linked with worried, sad or angry feelings.
Why body signals?	Some children enjoy reading and can be made to feel more involved. However, this can slow the session down. Briefly discuss how an awareness of your body signals can prevent you losing control and help you make better choices.
Types of body signals	Children are asked to report if they have ever experienced these sensations. This helps normalize the sensations related to anxiety.
Your own body signals	Children can show their drawings and share one or two body signals that they experience with the group. It can be important for children to notice how everyone is different and that is OK. Names given for body signals can be completely made up so long as they make sense to the individual child. For example the 'fuzzy wuzzy' feeling in my head or the 'wham bam whizzy' feeling in my tummy. Labelling body sensations is far more important than the quality of the drawings. 'Stick men' are fine.
What did your body do?	This exercise helps children become aware and name their (sometimes uncomfortable) physical sensations related to their feelings. Children are encouraged to feed back one or two sensations they have identified. Many children may not be aware that other children experience similar sensations when stressed. This can be shared with the group.

Personal alarms   Helps children see that body signals associated with anxiety are intended to help us cope. They have a useful function. It may be useful for children to see that the body signals or physical sensations are exactly the same regardless of whether they are worried something bad will happen or if the bad thing actually takes place (the fear of something is sometimes more scary than the reality).

Stay cool and take it easy   This relaxation exercise is aimed at helping children become aware of physical sensations and changes within their body. If you wish you can read from the text word for word. Alternatively, shorten or change the text to suit your group and time frame.

Or

Experiment 3.1   It is important to check that children do not suffer with medical conditions (such as severe asthma) before taking part in this exercise. Some children may connect this experiment with uncomfortable experiences of PE at school or perhaps a time in the past when they felt very anxious. Some children may be reluctant to take part in this activity. They can be invited to watch.

Experiment 3.2   Children should be encouraged to describe the differences between the two experiments. The aim is not necessarily to encourage children to use the strategies in Experiments 3.1 or 3.2 to calm themselves down when anxious (although both may reduce symptoms in the short term) but merely to create an awareness of body sensations and to normalize these experiences.

Home Activity 3: Body watching   Children are encouraged to observe others' body signals as a home activity. The aim of this activity is to further increase awareness and normalize (sometimes uncomfortable) body sensations.

Long session

Can include 'Tense and floppy game' and 'What did your body do?'. Also include both 'Stay cool and take it easy' and Experiments 3.1 and 3.2. In the short session there is too little time for all these exercises. Even in a long session you may consider that there is a lot to cover. Time permitting, children can also be encouraged to do some fun exercises at the beginning of the session such as running on the spot, playing tag, etc. Ask them what they notice in their bodies (heart rate increases, heavy breathing, etc.). What do they notice when looking at each other? In addition, videos/DVDs or pictures can be shown and children encouraged to guess how characters are feeling from looking at their body signals.

Notes

Experiments 3.1 and 3.2 are aimed at helping children become aware of their physiology and body signals. It may also be useful to help children explore the effects of changing their physiology on the way they feel emotionally. Children can conclude what they like about the exercises and their thoughts can be discussed openly in the group. For example, 'What was different about the two experiments?' 'What do the experiments teach us about our body signals?' 'Does this have a link with anxious feelings?' Some group facilitators running short sessions may seek advice about including 'Stay cool and take it easy' or Experiments 3.1 and 3.2. As a guide, although both exercises are intended to increase children's awareness of body signals, research suggests progressive muscle relaxation ('Stay cool and take it easy') is more useful for generalized anxiety (ongoing worries about 'everything and everyone'). However, Experiments 3.1 and 3.2 have been reported to be more fun. A greater contrast between body tension and relaxation is also observed by the children.

Tense and floppy game

The game is played like musical statues without music. The group members run around the room. When asked to 'tense' they stop running and assume a tense position. When the facilitator shouts 'floppy' the group assume a relaxed position.

List what you noticed when your body became tense	List what you noticed when your body became floppy

This game helps us:

- learn about the difference between tense and relaxed (floppy)
- become more aware of the physical changes in our bodies.

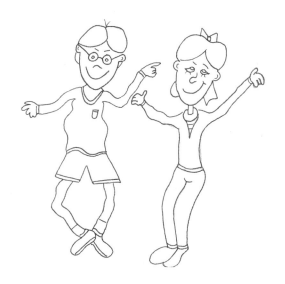

Why body signals?

Another important cool connection is learning how to identify and listen to your body signals. Our bodies are changing all the time, minute by minute throughout each day, depending on how we feel. You are probably unaware of these changes unless you experience a very strong feeling such as fear or anger. Thousands of years ago when we lived in caves people had to fight to survive. Cavemen didn't know any other way. They may have been threatened by wild animals who wanted to eat them or maybe someone had stolen their food or taken their home.

Today we are rarely attacked by wild animals. Instead we more often feel threatened by other human beings and what they may think of us. For example, 'Am I too fat or too thin?', 'I can't do the work at school', 'Will I fail my exams?', 'What will happen if I do?' Although these fears are not life or death threats our bodies don't always know the difference so we react in much the same way our cavemen ancestors reacted when wild animals attacked them.

Uncomfortable feelings such as anger or fear send strong signals or messages to all parts of the body to help prepare us to fight or run away from danger. This is sometimes called the fight-or-flight response. Suddenly hundreds of changes take place inside our bodies and we become 'pumped up' and ready for action. Our hearts pound faster, giving energy to our muscles, and we become tense and strong. Within a split second we can be ready to start a fight or run for our lives.

During this session we are going to become more aware of our body signals and the connections between them and our feelings. Recognizing and naming body signals will help us make choices about what action to take. It may also help prevent our feelings spiralling out of control like a racing car on the motorway without any brakes.

Unaware of body signals

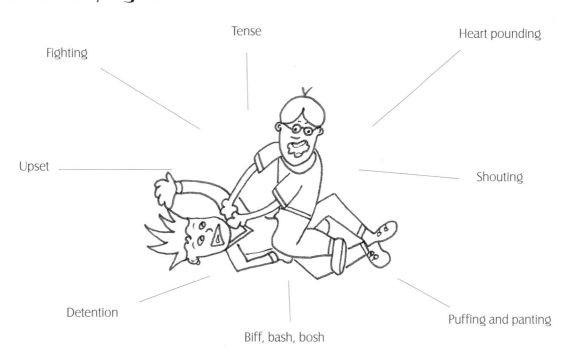

Tense

Heart pounding

Fighting

Upset

Shouting

Detention

Puffing and panting

Biff, bash, bosh

Aware of body signals

Body signals
My heart is pounding
My arms are tense

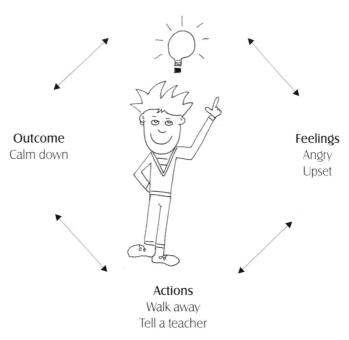

Outcome
Calm down

Feelings
Angry
Upset

Actions
Walk away
Tell a teacher

Types of body signals

It's important to learn the cool connections between your body signals when you are scared or worried.

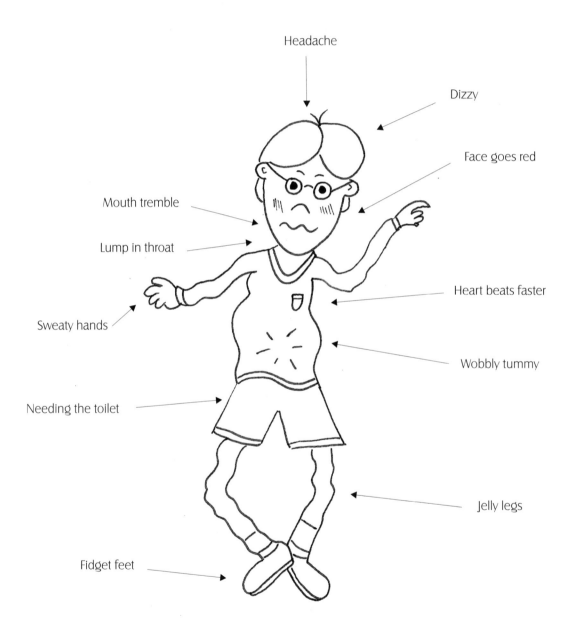

Headache

Dizzy

Face goes red

Mouth tremble

Lump in throat

Heart beats faster

Sweaty hands

Wobbly tummy

Needing the toilet

Jelly legs

Fidget feet

Your own body signals

Draw your own body in the box below showing your body signals when you are scared or worried. Everyone is different so your signals may be different from other people in your group.

What did your body do?

Draw yourself as a stick person and show with labels what happened to your body at a time you felt the following feelings:

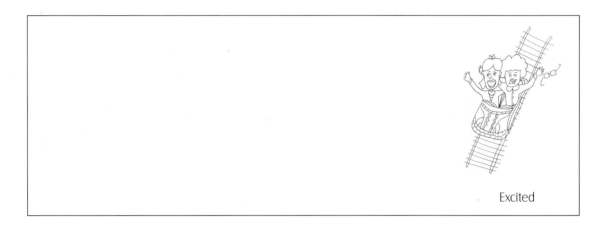

Excited

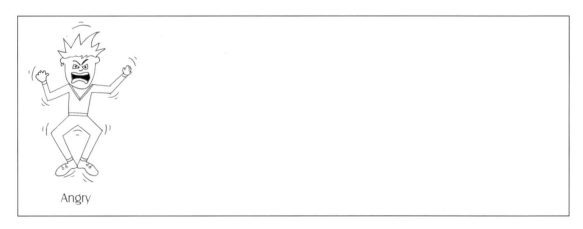

Angry

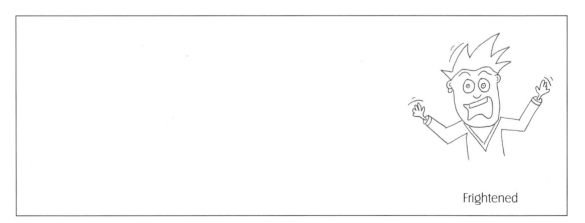

Frightened

Personal alarms

We all experience body signals. These signals are like a personal alarm inside us preparing our bodies for action. Our bodies quickly become pumped up and ready to fight or take flight and run away quickly. If you think back to a time when you felt upset or worried you may have noticed your body change. Here are some of the changes and the possible reasons for them.

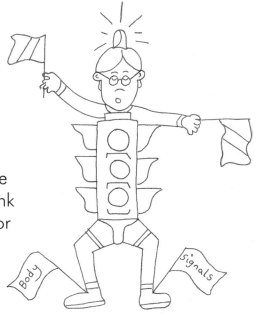

Body signals	Possible reasons
Sweating Needing the toilet	The body needs to lose fluids so it is lighter and you can run away or fight faster.
Breathing quickly/heavily	Your heart and lungs need more oxygen so that blood can be pumped to your muscles quickly, ready for action.
Numb or tingling hands and feet Dizziness Wobbly feelings	Blood rushes away from your hands and feet to the lungs and main muscles in your body so that you are stronger and can fight or take flight better.
Tense muscles Heart beating fast	The blood needs to be pumped round your body faster. Tense muscles make you more powerful and look more scary to an attacker.

If we did not experience body signals we would not be aware of pain or physical pleasure. We could even do our bodies some serious damage. Think, for example, what might happen if you kept walking on a broken leg or felt no pain after a serious bang on the head. Doctors would be very stuck working out what was wrong. We would not be able to tell the doctor which part of our bodies needed treatment.

The main job of body signals is to tell our brains what is happening in our bodies so that we can keep ourselves safe. Body signals themselves are always intended to be helpful. They are never bad or harmful. They are just body signals (headache, dizziness, shaking, etc.). However, the meaning we attach to these signals can often make us feel that we are in more danger than we really are. For example, you hear a noise downstairs while you are asleep in bed. You think someone is breaking in. When you go to look you find that it is only the cat coming in through the cat flap.

List the body signals that you may have if you are lying in bed at night and you think there is a burglar downstairs in your house.

```
+------------------------------------------------------------------+
|                                                                  |
|                                                                  |
|                                                                  |
|                                                                  |
+------------------------------------------------------------------+
```

List the body signals you may have if you go downstairs and there really is a burglar walking around in your house.

```
+------------------------------------------------------------------+
|                                                                  |
|                                                                  |
|                                                                  |
+------------------------------------------------------------------+
```

What do you notice about the body signals in the above situations?

```
+------------------------------------------------------------------+
|                                                                  |
|                                                                  |
|                                                                  |
+------------------------------------------------------------------+
```

Stay cool and take it easy

Today we're going to try some exercises to help us become more aware of our body signals and the physical changes that take place when we tense and relax. Exercises like these can help you learn to relax when you are feeling uptight or get those butterfly feelings in your stomach. They're also quite clever because you can learn how to do some of them without anyone really noticing.

In order for you to get the best feelings from these exercises, there are some rules you must follow. First, you must do exactly what I say, even if it seems kind of silly. Second, you must pay attention to your bodies and to how your muscles feel when they are tight and when they are loose and relaxed. Third, you must practise. The more you practise, the more relaxed you can become. Before we start, get as comfortable as you can in your chair. Sit back, put both feet on the floor, and just let your arms hang loose. Now close your eyes and don't open them until I say to. Remember to follow the instructions very carefully, try hard, and pay attention to your body signals.

Hands and arms

Pretend you have a whole lemon in your left hand. Now squeeze it hard. Try to squeeze all the juice out. Feel the tightness in your hand and arm as you squeeze. Now drop the lemon. Notice how your muscles feel when they are relaxed. Take another lemon and squeeze. Try to squeeze this one harder than you did the first one. That's right. Really hard. Now drop the lemon and relax. See how much better your hand and arm feel when they are relaxed. Once again, take a lemon in your left hand and squeeze all the juice out.

Don't leave a single drop. Squeeze hard. Good. Now relax and let the lemon fall from your hand. (Repeat the process for the right hand and arm.)

Arms and shoulders

Pretend you are a furry, lazy cat. You want to stretch. Stretch your arms out in front of you. Raise them up high over your head. Right back. Feel the pull in your shoulders. Stretch higher. Now just let your arms drop back to your side. Okay, let's stretch again. Stretch your arms out in front of you. Raise them over your head. Pull them back, pull hard. Now let them drop quickly. Good. Notice how your shoulders feel more relaxed. This time let's stretch really hard. Try to touch the ceiling. Stretch your arms way out in front of you. Raise them way up high over your head. Push them way, way back. Notice the tension and pull in your arms and shoulders. Hold tight. Great. Now let them drop very quickly and feel how good it is to be relaxed.

Jaw

You have a giant jawbreaker bubble gum in your mouth. It's very hard to chew. Bite down on it. Hard! Let your neck muscles help you. Now relax. Just let your jaw hang loose. Notice how good it feels just to let your jaw drop. Okay, let's tackle that jawbreaker again now. Bite down. Hard! Try to squeeze it out between your teeth. That's good. You're really tearing that gum up. Now relax again. Just let your jaw drop off your face. It feels good just to let go and not have to fight that bubble gum.

Face and nose

Here comes a really annoying fly. He has landed on your nose. Try to get him off without using your hands. That's right, wrinkle up your nose. Make as many wrinkles in your nose as you can. Scrunch your nose up real hard. Good. You've chased him away. Now you can relax your nose. Oops, here he comes back again. Right back in the middle of your nose. Wrinkle up your nose again. Shoo him off. Wrinkle it up hard. Hold it just as tight as you can. Okay, he flew away. You can relax your face. Notice that when you scrunch up your nose your cheeks and your mouth and your forehead and your eyes all help you, and they get tight too. So when you relax your nose, your whole body relaxes too, and that feels good. Oh-oh. This time that old fly has come back, but this time he's on your forehead. Make lots of wrinkles. Try to catch him between all those wrinkles. Hold it tight, now. Okay, you can let go. He's gone for good. Now you can just relax. Let your face go smooth, no wrinkles anywhere. Your face feels nice and smooth and relaxed.

Stomach

Imagine you can see a cute baby elephant. He's not watching where he's going. He doesn't see you lying in the grass, and he's about to step on your stomach. Don't move. You don't have time to get out of the way. Just get ready for him. Make your stomach very hard. Tighten up your stomach muscles real tight. Hold it. It looks like he is going the other way. You can relax now. Let your stomach go soft. Let it be as relaxed as you can. That feels so much better. Oops, he's coming this way again. Get ready. Tighten up your stomach. Really hard. If he steps on you when your stomach is hard, it won't hurt. Make your stomach into a rock. Okay, he's moving away again. You can relax now. Kind of settle down, get comfortable, and relax. Notice the difference between a tight stomach and a relaxed one. That's how we want to feel – nice and loose and relaxed.

Legs

Now pretend that you are standing barefoot in a large dirty mud puddle. Squish your toes down deep into the mud. Try to get your feet down to the bottom of the mud puddle. You'll probably need your legs to help you push. Push down, spread your toes apart, feel the mud squish up between your toes. Now step out of the mud puddle. Relax your feet. Let your toes go loose and feel how nice it is to be relaxed. Back into the mud puddle. Squish your toes down. Let your leg muscles help push your feet down. Push your feet. Hard. Try to squeeze that puddle dry. Okay. Come back out now. Relax your feet, relax your legs, relax your toes. It feels so good to be relaxed. No tenseness anywhere. You feel kind of warm and tingly.

Conclusion

Stay as relaxed as you can. Let your whole body go limp and feel all your muscles relaxed. In a few minutes I will ask you to open your eyes, and that will be the end of this practice session. As you go through the day, remember how good it feels to be relaxed. Sometimes you have to make yourself tighter before you can be relaxed, just as we did in these exercises. Practise these exercises every day to get more and more relaxed. A good time to practise is at night after you have gone to bed and the lights are out and you won't be disturbed. It will help you get to sleep. Then, when you are really a good relaxer, you can help yourself relax at school. Just remember the elephant or the jawbreaker or the mud puddle and you can do our exercises and nobody will know. Today is a good day, and you are ready to feel very relaxed. You've worked hard and it feels good to work hard. Very slowly, now, open your eyes and wiggle your muscles around a little. Very good.

Adapted from Koeppen, A.S. (1974) 'Relaxation Training for Children.' *Elementary School Guidance and Counseling, 9*, 14–21.

Experiment 3.1

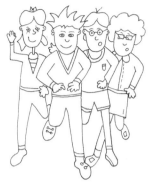

In the following exercise we are going to experiment and make cool connections by becoming more aware of the effects of physical exercise on our bodies.

Stand up and run on the spot for between 30 seconds and one minute before completing the boxes below.

What body signals/sensations are you aware of right now?

What do you notice about your heart rate and your breathing?

What do you think might happen if you kept doing this exercise?

Write about a time that you have experienced these body signals before.

Experiment 3.2

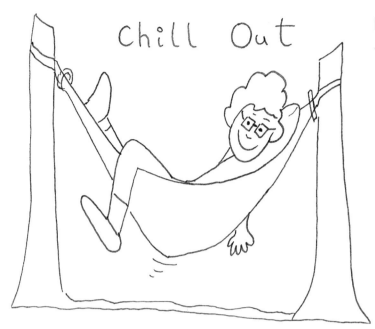

Breathe slowly and deeply, counting in–2–3 and out–2–3. Imagine you are on a sunny beach with the waves gently lapping against the sea shore. Breathe deeply for about a minute. Let your stomach rise and fall. Imagine your stomach is like the tides of the sea. As you breathe out slowly imagine the tide coming in again like a wave.

What body signals/sensations are you aware of right now?

What do you notice about your heart rate and your breathing?

What do you think might happen if you kept doing this exercise?

Write about a time that you have experienced these body signals before.

In Experiments 3.1 and 3.2 you were encouraged to become more aware of your body signals. Write anything that you noticed about the experiments in the box below. Have you learned anything that might help you next time you feel scared or worried?

Home Activity 3: Body watching

Red face (blushing)	Dry mouth (lip smacking)	Sweating	Tense body (stiff)
Shaking	Heavy breathing (panting)	Choking/ retching (like being sick)	Tearful (crying/ laughing)
Screwed-up face (snarling/pain)	Clenched fists	Heart pounding (see their pulse)	Cheeks puffed (like smiling)

Watch your friends, family and teachers this week and see if you can make cool connections by spotting all the body signals written above. Write them in the boxes below:

Body signal	Child = C Adult = A	What are they doing at the time?
Example: Red face	A	Shouting at a group of naughty children in school

SESSION 4: Identifying Thoughts

Aims and objectives

- Help identify thoughts.
- Learn the effect our thinking has on our feelings and actions.

Materials

Chairs, pencils, small tub or box for folded paper in exercise on page 104.

Agenda and tips for running the session

Exercises in bold in the left-hand column should be included in both long and short sessions. Other exercises are optional and can be included in groups where there is more time. Many fun activities/games are included as optional. Despite sometimes being short of time it is important not to cut all the 'fun' out of the programme or you will lose the children's enthusiasm.

Short session

EXERCISE	COMMENTS
Feedback	Welcome the children and share agenda for session with group. Obtain brief feedback about the children's week.
Review Home Activity 3	Group facilitators collect home activities from Session 3 to explore in more detail after this session and return the following week (Session 5) or at the end of the programme. Questions may be asked about the previous week's homework.
Thought whisper game	Fun way to demonstrate how thoughts can be misinterpreted. Game works best if the facilitator makes up the first short sentence to avoid confusion.
About thoughts	Some children enjoy reading and can be made to feel more involved. However, this can slow the session down.
Fill in the thought bubbles	Children begin to identify thoughts. Each child can be asked to feed back to the group one or two of the thoughts he or she has associated with the different characters on the page.
Different thoughts	Children write different thoughts about themselves than those they consider other children have about them. It is likely that the thoughts children write about other children are closely linked to thoughts/beliefs that they have about themselves. However, this cannot be taken as fact and if appropriate this may need to be checked out with individual children. Children can be asked to feed back to the group one or two different thoughts they have identified. It is useful to help the group identify how some children think in similar ways while others think quite differently. There is no right or wrong way of thinking. Thoughts are just thoughts!

Thought–feeling cool connections	Shows the connection between thoughts and feelings. May help children begin to empathize with how others feel when children are cruel or say unkind things. It is useful to share with the group that children sometimes say unkind 'nasty' things to themselves in their own thoughts, for example 'you're stupid or weird'. Children can be questioned about how they feel inside when they think these unpleasant things about themselves. It is important that children do not write their names on the paper or personalize their unhelpful thoughts about any members of the group.
Catching thoughts example	Read page to the children and ask what they think about these examples. Encourage the children to make connections between the way the children look, feel and think. For example, 'How do you think the children in the examples are feeling?' 'How would you feel if you had these thoughts?'
Catching thoughts	Children are encouraged to share their thoughts with the group but should not be pressurized to do so. A comment about confidentiality within the group may help children disclose more personal information.
Home Activity 4: Catching thoughts	This encourages children to practise catching thoughts. Just catching thoughts can make a significant difference to the way they feel. Catching specific thoughts helps children develop awareness and begin to validate their feelings.

Long session

More time can be spent on feedback. Include 'Thought whisper game'. Children can be shown comics with examples of thought bubbles. Some self-help videos/DVDs show examples of thoughts which can be shared with the children. For example, the videos associated with the Coping Cat Series (Kendall) which can be obtained from Workbook Publishing (www.workbookpublishing.com). Some films also provide excellent examples of thoughts, for example *What Women Want*, in which Mel

Gibson, who acts as a sales rep, has an accident and is suddenly able to hear the thoughts of women. It can be noted how being able to hear these thoughts changes his feelings and behaviour towards the women around him. (As this film is rated age 15, consent should be obtained from parents, even if only showing a censored clip to this age group of children.) In some sessions we have given children a cut-out of a famous character (Donald Duck, Superman, etc.) and played a guessing game, matching the different thoughts they may have about themselves. For example, 'What's up Doc' and 'I love carrots' would match with Bugs Bunny, and 'I'm always on the web' or 'I am such a superhero' would match Spiderman, etc. This game is good fun and helps children identify with the fact that different people have different thoughts about themselves.

Notes

The exercises in this session aim to help children become aware of their thoughts. Children are informed that thoughts can also be images or 'pictures in their heads'. Some children may choose to draw their thoughts, which is fine, although not much room is provided in the text boxes.

Thought whisper game

- All children sit in a circle.

- One group member whispers a short sentence or thought to the person sitting next to them.

- This person in turn whispers what they heard to the next person, and so on round the circle.

- The last person announces what they heard.

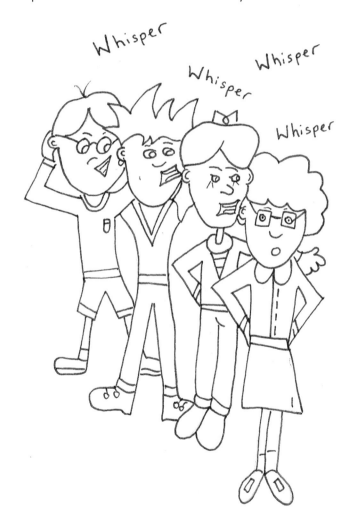

- This game provides a fun way to show how thoughts can get misinterpreted.

- People tend to hear what they want to hear rather than what has actually been said.

About thoughts

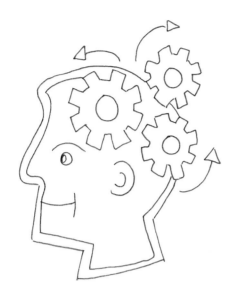

Everybody has thoughts, and this includes children, adults, and even babies. Thoughts go on all the time in our heads. Sometimes they are like words or sentences and sometimes they are in the form of pictures, as in our dreams. We have thoughts about ourselves such as 'I'm so fantastic', thoughts about other people, for example 'I don't like her, she's horrid', and thoughts about the things around us, like 'my school is so cool' or 'the world can be a dangerous place'. Everyone is different so everyone has different thoughts.

The cool connections about our thoughts are that they make a difference to how we feel and what we do. Some of the thoughts we have can make us feel angry, sad or worried. For example, 'I'm ugly, no-one likes me' or 'I'm never going to get picked for the team'. Other thoughts can make us feel happy or excited, such as 'I'm the cleverest in the school, everyone loves me' or 'I'm going to the fair tonight with my mates'.

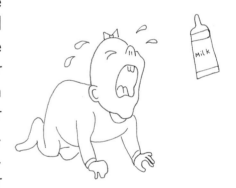

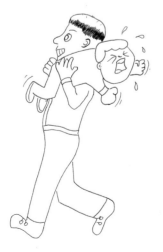

There are many people who believe that there are good and bad thoughts. However, the truth is that thoughts are just thoughts – it's what you *do* that makes the difference. In the following example both Jack and Katie have angry thoughts. In your view which child is most likely to get into trouble?

Jack felt so angry that he thought about hitting his little sister but he decided to go for a run instead.

Katie thought her brother was horrid so she broke his favourite computer game.

Sometimes we are aware of our thinking but a lot of the time our thoughts go unnoticed. By stopping and listening to your thoughts you can find out a lot about yourself and your feelings. In today's session we will be learning more about thoughts and how to catch them so that we can find out more about ourselves.

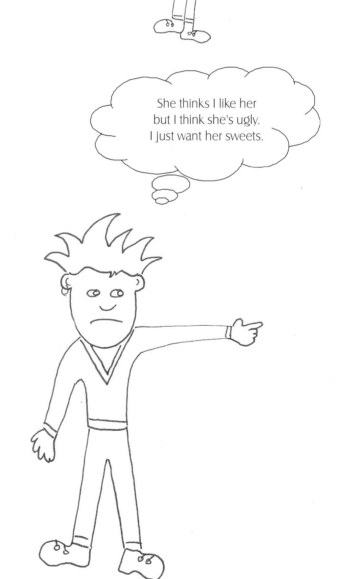

Fill in the thought bubbles

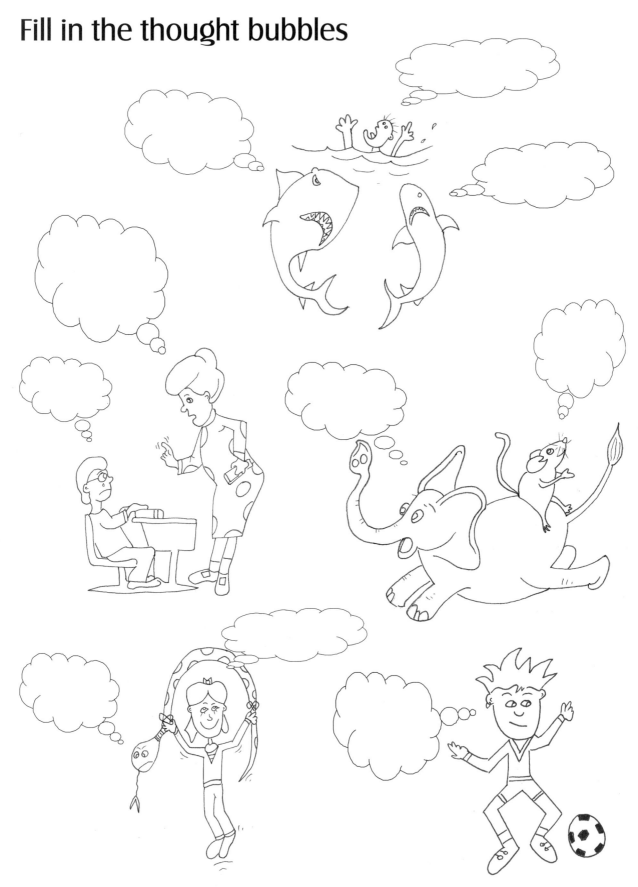

Different thoughts

All of us have different thoughts running through our minds all the time. Some of these thoughts make us feel happy inside while others make us feel angry, sad or scared. Make cool connections by writing some of the thoughts other children may have in the different situations below:

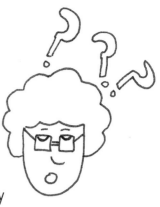

Thoughts about themselves

Happy thoughts	Sad, worried or angry thoughts

Their school

Happy thoughts	Sad, worried or angry thoughts

Their home

Happy thoughts	Sad, worried or angry thoughts

Thought–feeling cool connections

- Group members sit in a circle and each is given two small pieces of paper.

- On one piece of paper they write something that would make someone else feel good about themselves (for example: 'I like your smile' or 'you are good fun to be with').

- On the other paper they write something mean or nasty like a bully might say (for example: 'you're horrid' or 'you are so ugly').

- All the paper messages are folded and placed *anonymously* in a tub or box.

- Group members take two random pieces of paper from the tub.

- Each child reads the paper messages one at a time facing the person next to them.

- The group are asked to report how they would feel and what they would do if the statements were said to them.

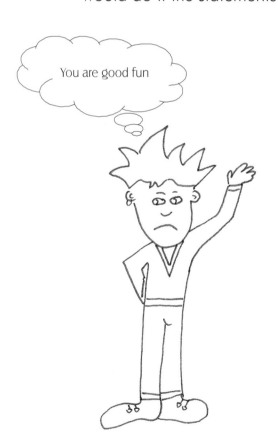

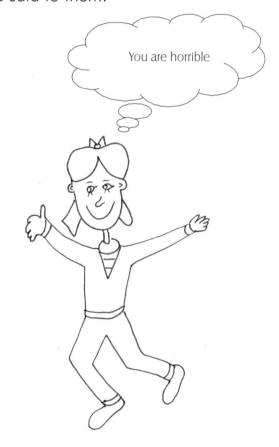

Catching thoughts example

Now that you have learned the cool connections about thoughts and feelings look at the examples below showing Katie and Harry's thoughts and feelings in different situations. Notice how their thoughts seem to affect the way they look and feel.

What happened? Mrs Jones my English teacher told me to read out in front of the whole class.

How does my face look?

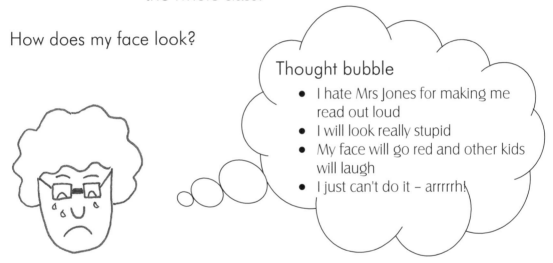

Thought bubble

- I hate Mrs Jones for making me read out loud
- I will look really stupid
- My face will go red and other kids will laugh
- I just can't do it – arrrrrh!

What happened? Fred Bloggs pushed me in the playground and I fell over.

How does my face look?

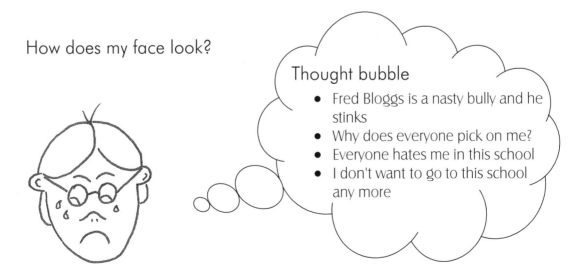

Thought bubble

- Fred Bloggs is a nasty bully and he stinks
- Why does everyone pick on me?
- Everyone hates me in this school
- I don't want to go to this school any more

Catching thoughts

Make cool connections between your thoughts and feelings. Next to 'What happened?' write something from the past or present that has made you feel unhappy, angry or scared. In the thoughts box write or draw the thoughts you had about this. Finally, under 'How does my face look?', draw how the thoughts made you feel. If you cannot think of an example for yourself make one up about a friend or member of your family. Good luck!!

What happened? _

How does my face look?

Thought bubble

What happened? _

How does my face look?

Thought bubble

Home Activity 4: Catching thoughts

In the last session we learned about catching thoughts. Here is another chance to practise. Next to 'What happened?' write something that has happened to you that made you feel unhappy, angry or scared. In the thoughts box write or draw the thoughts you had about this. Finally, under 'How does my face look?', draw what your face may have looked like at the time. If you prefer you can make up an example about a friend or a member of your family.

What happened? _

How does my face look?

Thought bubble

What happened? _

How does my face look?

Thought bubble

SESSION 5: The Connections between Thoughts, Feelings, Body Signals and Actions

Aims and objectives

- Understand the links between thoughts, feelings, body signals and actions.
- Pull together the other sessions in the programme so far.
- See how a change in either our thinking, feeling, body signals or actions can affect the other connections.
- Notice similarities and differences between yourself and others in the group.

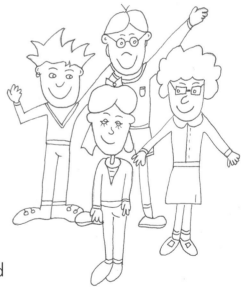

Materials

Chairs, pencils, a hoop, large paper labels with thoughts, feelings, body signals and actions written on separate pieces of paper for 'Cool Connections game'.

Agenda and tips for running the session

Exercises in bold in the left-hand column should be included in both long and short sessions. Other exercises are optional and can be included in groups where there is more time. Many fun activities/games are included as optional. Despite sometimes being short of time it is important not to cut all the 'fun' out of the programme or you will lose the children's enthusiasm.

Short session

EXERCISE	COMMENTS
Feedback	Welcome the children and share agenda for session with group. Obtain brief feedback about the children's week.
Review Home Activity 4	Children can briefly show work. Facilitators collect home activities to explore in more detail after the session and return the following week or at the end of the programme.
Hoops	Fun activity to help children warm up in session.
The Zog from Zen	This story is aimed at helping children begin to understand the cognitive model (links between thoughts, feelings, physical sensations and behaviour). Some children enjoy reading and can be made to feel more involved. However, this can slow the session down.
Your actions	Helps children become more self-aware by making connections between their feelings and their actions.
Different cool connections	This section can be read to the children or they can be asked to read this to themselves and then feed back to the group.
Cool connections example	Group facilitator shares example on page 119. The group can be asked if they would have similar or different feelings, body signals, thoughts, etc. to the child in the example.
My cool connections	If children cannot identify a time when they felt frightened or sad they can either make it up or use a time when a parent or friend felt this way. There are no right or wrong answers. Children can choose to share their examples or keep them private.

Cool connections game	Use the sentences listed on page 123 for the game or make up your own.
Home Activity 5a: Quick quiz	This helps reinforce the cool connections learned so far. It increases facilitators' awareness of how well group members are beginning to understand the cognitive model (links between thoughts and feelings).
Home Activity 5b: Cool connections	It is useful to inform children that their home activity work is kept confidential and will not be shared with the group without their consent.

Long session

More time can be spent on each exercise. Include the 'Hoops' and the 'Cool connections' games. To illustrate further the way our thoughts and feelings are linked it can be useful to show a video/DVD clip of how someone's behaviour changes when he or she gets new or different information. With boys I often use a clip from *The Karate Kid* where the young karate student is angry with his teacher for making him paint the fence, sand the floor, and wax the car. His mood and behaviour completely change when he learns that he has been learning karate techniques all along.

Notes

The exercises in this session are about gaining an awareness of thoughts, feelings, body signals and actions, and the connections between them. It is more beneficial if children are prepared to share their own material and write personal thoughts, feelings, etc. in the boxes provided in the session, but this is not essential. Merely becoming aware of thoughts, feelings, body signals and actions, and the connections between them (the cognitive model), will help children develop their own emotional literacy skills. With practice children can begin to label their own feelings and gain a better awareness of the emotional experiences of others.

Hoops

Group members stand in a circle. Each child links hands or arms with the children either side of him or her. One child places a hoop around themselves. The object of the exercise is to move the hoop from person to person right round the circle without using hands and breaking the connection between the children in the circle.

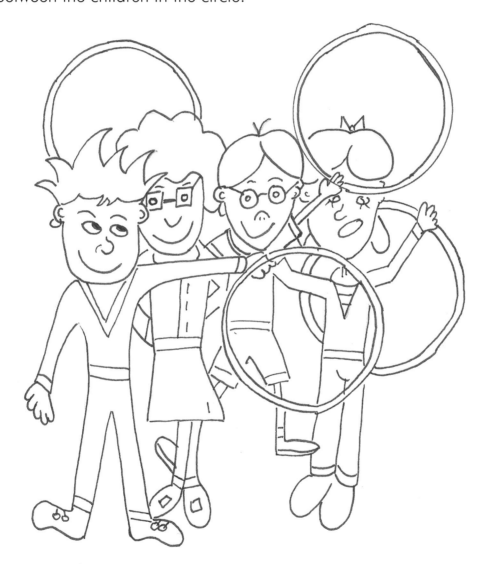

This game indicates that:

- problem solving is easier with the help of others
- when things are connected if one part moves it affects the other parts.

The Zog from Zen

In this session we are going to look at the cool way that your thoughts, feelings, body signals and actions are all connected. Listen to the story below.

The Zog is an alien from outer space who lives on the planet Zen. One day he woke up feeling excited because it was his birthday. The Zog's body felt tingly and he noticed a warm fuzzy feeling in his tummy. He said to himself, 'Today will be great because I'm having a party. All my Zen friends are coming. I love birthdays.' He quickly jumped out of bed, put on his Zen clothes and went off to the party at the Zen village hall.

Notice how the Zog's thoughts, feelings, body signals and actions are all connected. One part cannot move without the other.

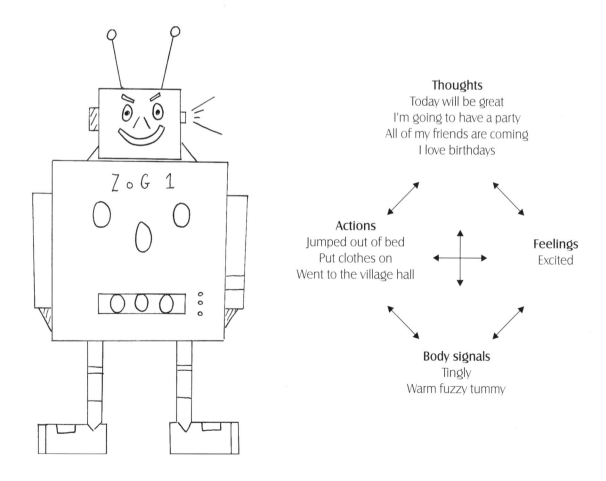

Thoughts
Today will be great
I'm going to have a party
All of my friends are coming
I love birthdays

Actions
Jumped out of bed
Put clothes on
Went to the village hall

Feelings
Excited

Body signals
Tingly
Warm fuzzy tummy

The time came for the party to begin but no alien friends arrived. The Zog looked out of the window but he could not see any of his Zen friends arriving. As time went by the Zog began to feel sad and worried. His mouth felt dry and his throat felt like there was a lump in it. The Zog's tummy started to turn over and over and his alien heart pounded in his chest. He thought, 'What shall I do? I've been forgotten', 'My alien friends don't like me', and 'I'm like Billy No-mates'. The Zog sat down, put his head in his hands and cried. Can you work out what goes in each box?

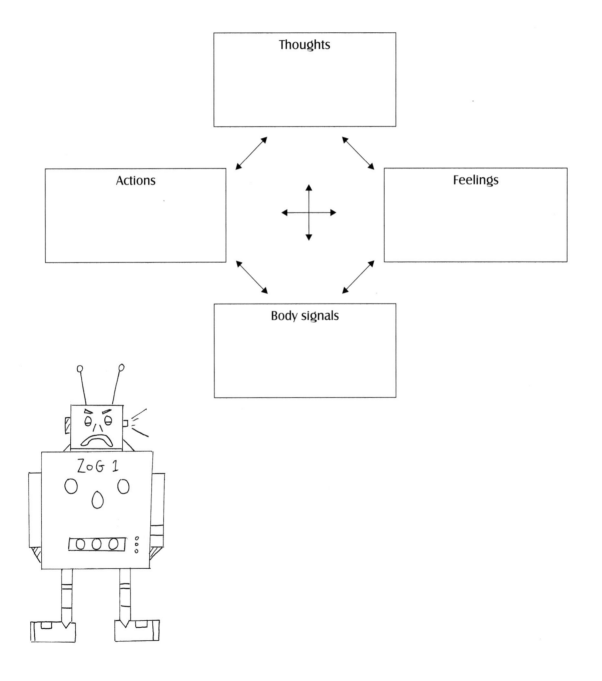

The Zog's thoughts, feelings, body signals and actions had all changed and become like a vicious cycle. The more worried and sad thoughts he had the more upset he felt.

After some time the Zog returned home. As he arrived he heard his Zen friends singing 'Happy Birthday' and calling his name. They had prepared a surprise party at his home. At this point the Zog's sad and worried feelings started to change. He became happy and overjoyed. His tummy became calm and his body was relaxed. His thoughts also changed: 'Everyone remembered me', 'My friends care about me' and 'I love birthdays'. The Zog laughed and jumped up and down with excitement.

Notice how the Zog's thoughts, feelings, body signals and actions all changed once again.

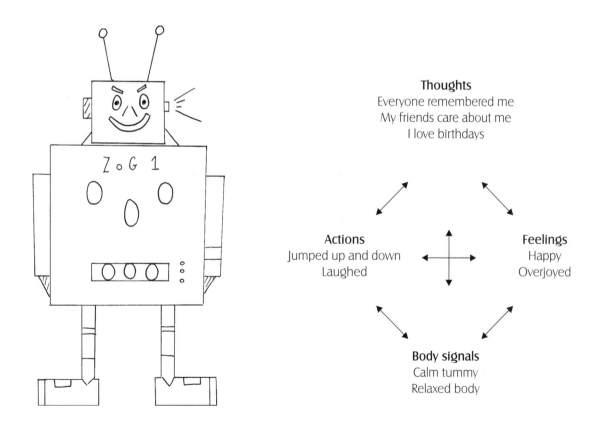

Thoughts
Everyone remembered me
My friends care about me
I love birthdays

Actions
Jumped up and down
Laughed

Feelings
Happy
Overjoyed

Body signals
Calm tummy
Relaxed body

Adapted from Friedberg, R.D. *et al.* (2001) 'Diamond Connections.' In *Therapeutic Exercises for Children: Guided Self-Discovery using Cognitive-Behavioral Techniques* (pp.8–11). Copyright 2001 Professional Resource Exchange, Inc., Sarasota, Fl. Adapted with permission.

Your actions

Sometimes when you feel sad you don't have as much fun doing the things you used to like doing. You give up on things faster, or get into more fights with family and friends. When you are scared you might have bad dreams or become more shy around people. You may also stay away from the things that scare you, for example dogs, school or lifts. List some of the cool connections between your actions and your scared and sad feelings.

Draw or write your actions or the things that you do when you are sad:

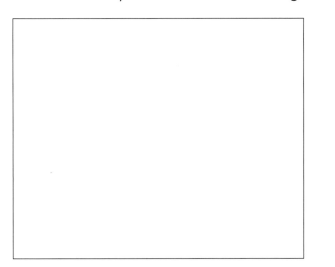

Draw or write your actions or the things that you do when you are scared:

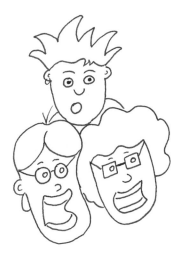

Different cool connections

Human beings can quickly change from one feeling to another, for example calm and happy to feeling angry, scared or stressed out. This is because we have a super-fast communication system in our brains which connects our thoughts, feelings, body signals and actions.

Situation

A child bumps into you in the school corridor. Notice how different people react to the same situation depending on their different thoughts and feelings.

Angry

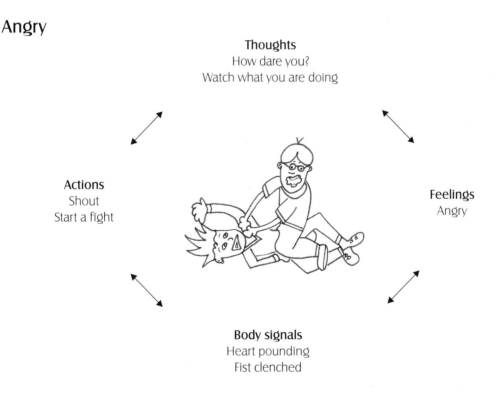

Thoughts
How dare you?
Watch what you are doing

Actions
Shout
Start a fight

Feelings
Angry

Body signals
Heart pounding
Fist clenched

Excited

Thoughts
Wow! Harry bumped into me
It's because he likes me

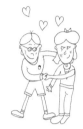

Actions
Smile sweetly
Laugh and joke

Feelings
Excited
Embarrassed

Body signals
Heart pounding
Face goes red
Butterflies

Worried

Thoughts
The poor boy
I need to help him

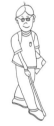

Actions
Offer to help
Ask if he's OK

Feelings
Worried
Concerned

Body signals
Stiff hands
Butterflies

Sad

Thoughts
I'm so stupid. No-one likes me
Other kids just knock me around

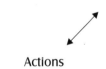

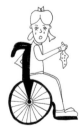

Actions
Avoid people
Stop going to school
Let kids pick on me

Feelings
Sad
Lonely

Body signals
Heart pounding
Fist clenched

Cool connections example

What happened?

My mum and dad were shouting at each other last night. Mum ended up walking out and slamming the door.

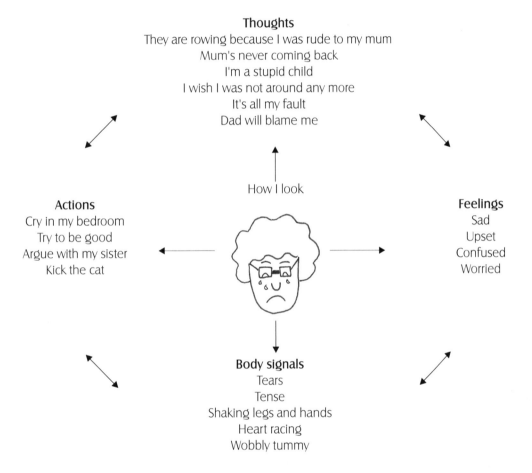

Thoughts
They are rowing because I was rude to my mum
Mum's never coming back
I'm a stupid child
I wish I was not around any more
It's all my fault
Dad will blame me

How I look

Actions
Cry in my bedroom
Try to be good
Argue with my sister
Kick the cat

Feelings
Sad
Upset
Confused
Worried

Body signals
Tears
Tense
Shaking legs and hands
Heart racing
Wobbly tummy

From the cycle above you can see that Katie is very upset about the row her parents had last night. Notice how her thoughts, feelings, body signals and actions are all connected with each other. Katie is clearly upset about her parents rowing. However, until she completed the boxes above, she was totally unaware of what thoughts and body signals were making her feel so unhappy and causing her to cry and lash out at others. Looking at the completed boxes has helped Katie to see the situation differently and explore her feelings more clearly.

My cool connections

Now it's your turn. First think of a time you were frightened and then a time you were sad before completing the boxes. Make cool connections by drawing how your face looked in the centre of each cycle.

I felt frightened when:

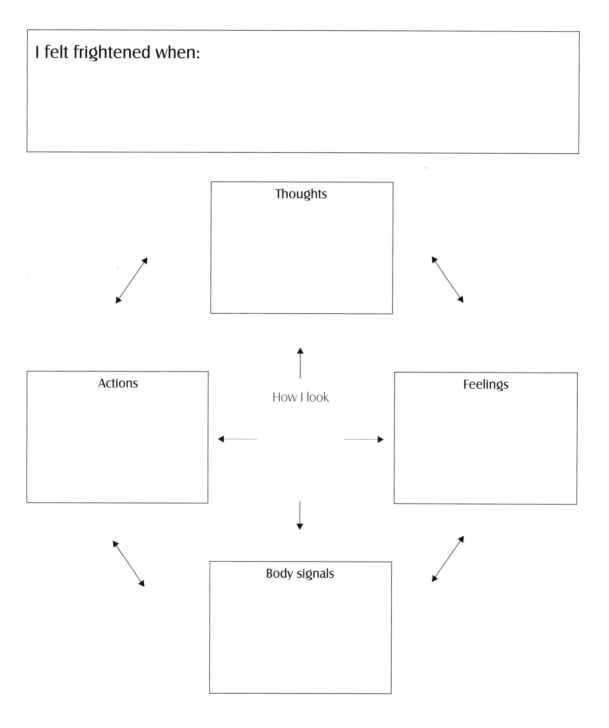

I felt sad when:

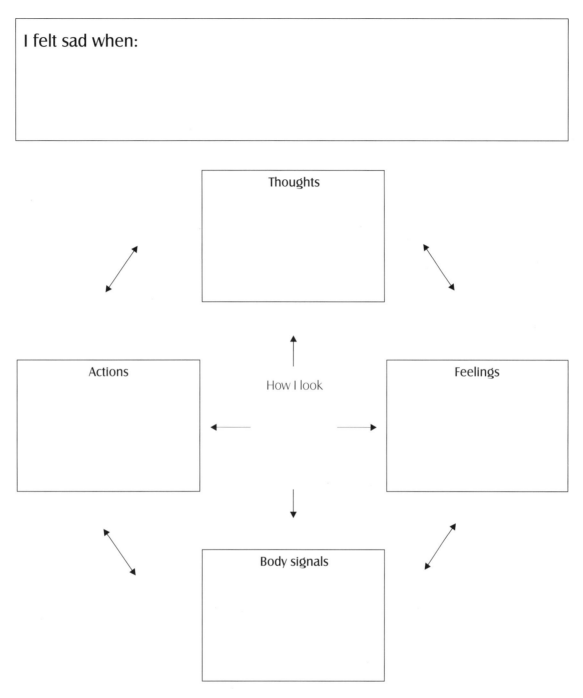

Cool connections game

The following game is a further example of how your thoughts, feelings, body signals and actions are all connected.

How to play

- Find four pieces of paper or card. On each separate sheet write one of the following words.

THOUGHTS   **FEELINGS**   **BODY SIGNALS**   **ACTIONS**

- Stick one piece of paper to each of the four walls in the room.
- Facilitator reads out the passage on the following page. When the group members recognize thoughts, feelings, body signals or actions from the sentences they must run to the associated part of the room. For example, if the facilitator reads 'Mary was feeling really sad' the group run to the area of the room marked 'feelings'.

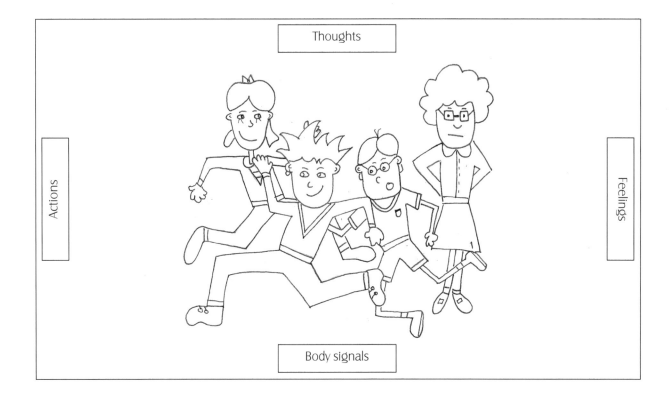

The game

- The Cool Connections Programme makes us feel so *happy*.

- Some boys at school took my lunch money and I thought, '*How dare they – I'm going to tell a teacher.*'

- I went to the dentist and looked up at the drill. My *heart started to pound in my chest*.

- The old lady saw a spider on the wall in her bedroom. She was so shocked that she *ran out of the room screaming*.

- The lion escaped from its cage at the zoo. I was so scared I started to *panic*.

- '*Help, help, help,*' thought the caretaker as he slipped on the wet floor.

- The girl stuck chewing gum on her chair at school. She started to feel quite *sick* when she noticed the head teacher looking at her.

- The boy *ran away* when he saw the bullies coming towards him.

- The girl found her maths test very *frustrating*.

- The children enjoyed the games so much that they thought, '*We'd like to play that again.*'

Home Activity 5a: Quick quiz

In the box below practise making cool connections by ticking whether the statements in the box on the left are thoughts, feelings, body signals or actions.

	Thought	Feeling	Body signal	Action
'I hate being away from my friends'				
Shaking				
Kicking a ball				
Tired				
'I really like pop music'				
'Oh no, here come those feelings again'				
Angry				
Sick				
Dizzy				
Climbing over the fence				
Frustrated				
'The teachers are so cool'				
Running				
Playing football				
'My fingers have gone tingly'				
Sweating				
'I love my clothes'				
Worried				
'It's driving me mad – I just can't cope'				
Upset				

Home Activity 5b: Cool connections

Notice a time this week when you have had a strong feeling and then complete the boxes below. This could be a time when you have felt worried, upset, angry or sad. Write briefly what happened in the box before completing your cool connections (for example, Harry bullied me at school, or my mum told me off). Draw what your face looked like in the centre of the boxes.

What has happened?

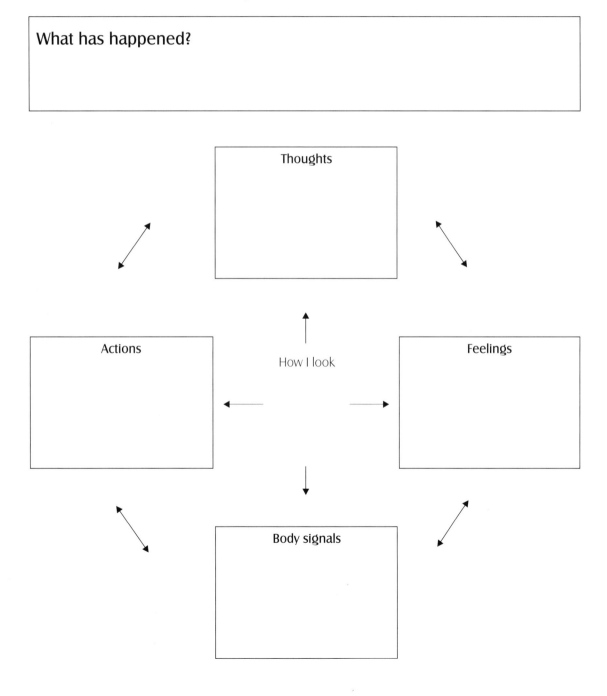

What has happened?

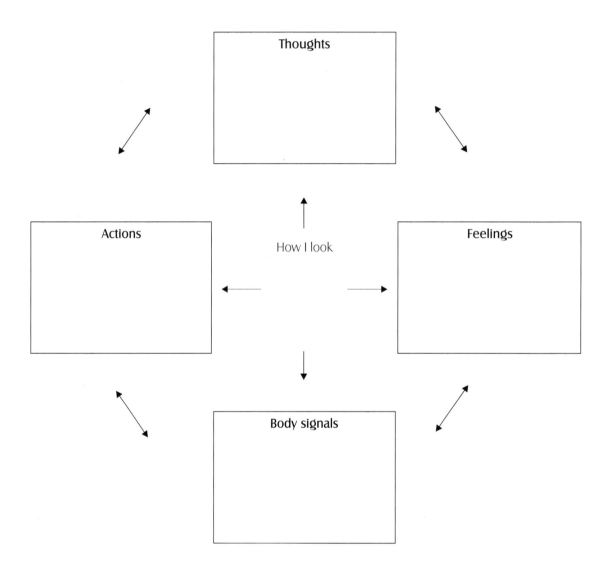

Thoughts

Actions

How I look

Feelings

Body signals

SESSION 6: Types of Thinking

Aims and objectives

- Learn that there are different ways of thinking and that these can affect how we feel and act.
- Learn questions which help us understand in more detail what is upsetting us.

Materials

Chairs, pencils, cap or hat for exercise on page 134 (not essential). Selection of hand or finger puppets.

Agenda and tips for running the session

Exercises in bold in the left-hand column should be included in both long and short sessions. Other exercises are optional and can be included in groups where there is more time. Many fun activities/ games are included as optional. Despite sometimes being short of time it is important not to cut all the 'fun' out of the programme or you will lose the children's enthusiasm.

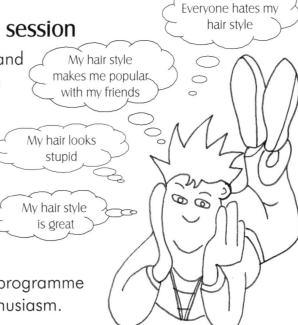

Everyone hates my hair style

My hair style makes me popular with my friends

My hair looks stupid

My hair style is great

Short session

EXERCISE	COMMENTS
Feedback	Welcome the children and share agenda for session with group. Obtain brief feedback from children's week.
Review Home Activities 5a and 5b	Children can briefly share their work. Facilitators collect home activities to explore in more detail after the session and return the following week or at the end of the programme.
'Get knotted'	Fun way to start the session. If children are reluctant to hold hands they can hold jumper/shirt sleeves or wrists.
The beautiful hag	Children are encouraged to feed back on the pictures. It is emphasized that there are no right or wrong answers. It is interesting how different children perceive the pictures. We have noticed that negative thinkers often see the old hag first and the two faces as aggressive. Children with a more positive outlook tend to observe the beautiful lady first and suggest seeing two lovers/friends.
Are you a Pollyanna?	Children are asked to volunteer a couple of the characters they have placed in each box. Children may also be asked in which box they would place themselves.
The gloomies	From this exercise we have noticed that children who feel unhappy about themselves are often particularly good at this exercise. A cap or hat can be worn by the gloomy thinker at the discretion of the facilitators.
Downward diggers	Children are encouraged to choose to read the different parts. You may wish to include puppets for this exercise.

My downward digger	Children find using puppets good fun and the children can hide behind the puppet characters they have chosen. Some facilitators may prefer not to use puppets or would rather use a different tool for the exercise. For example, children could dress up, wear different hats or draw the answers using speech bubbles. This exercise can sometimes make children feel low, especially if they connect the puppet's worry or upset with themselves. Other group members can be encouraged to offer support and/or help with this. See Notes on page 130.

Or

Helping hands	Some children may find difficulty identifying people they can trust to support them or find difficulty thinking of activities they enjoy doing. This can be an indicator that the child is experiencing low mood or depression. On these occasions facilitators should empathize with the individual and invite the other group members to offer their support. Following the group a network should be developed either by facilitators or teachers to provide support for the child. Buddy groups, school prefects or mentors can be useful here. Also children can be encouraged to get involved in inside or outside school/activity groups.
Wise worriers	This is a helpful exercise, especially in reducing generalized anxiety (when children seem to have ongoing worries about everything all of the time). When children struggle with this exercise it may highlight high levels of anxiety or difficulties with problem-solving. In some cases, thinking about themselves having these anxiety-provoking scenarios may feel too threatening. Instead, the child should be encouraged to write what a friend would do in the scenarios.
Home Activity 6: Eavesdropping	Children gain an awareness of different types of thinking. This can help normalize their own experiences and develop alternative ways of thinking.

Long session

Include 'Get knotted', 'Downward diggers', 'My downward digger', 'Helping hands' and 'Wise worriers'. More time can be spent with 'The gloomies' and 'Downward diggers'/'Helping hands' and 'Wise worriers'. Children can act out an example of a positive thinker or negative thinker. We found it useful to show a clip from the *Pollyanna* video/DVD. The children can be asked what they notice about the effect Pollyanna's 'Glad game' and general attitude to life have on the people around her.

Notes

We are not aiming to help children become positive thinkers instead of negative thinkers. Rather we are helping children to become aware of the effect different types of thinking can have on their feelings, body signals and actions. Children often have quite fixed 'black and white' ways of thinking. The first part of this session aims to introduce some 'shades of grey' and explore alternative ways of thinking about things. The 'Downward diggers' exercise is quite difficult and can cause children to become quite frustrated. However, the aim is to help children get to the heart of what is troubling them. Looking at the worst possible outcomes can help reduce anxieties in some children, while in others coping/problem-solving strategies are initiated. The 'Helping hands' and 'Wise worriers' exercises provide children with some basic ways to help cope with their fears and anxious thoughts. Some facilitators running short sessions may seek advice in choosing between 'Downward diggers' and 'Helping hands'/'Wise worriers'. As a guide the 'Downward diggers' exercise is a useful tool for children who are frequently upset or anxious but remain unclear regarding the thoughts/beliefs which are maintaining these feelings. 'Helping hands'/'Wise worriers' are useful for children who feel isolated or helpless and provide a useful strategy for coping with generalized anxiety or worries that feel 'out of control'.

'Get knotted'

- The group form a chain by holding hands or wrists.
- One end of the chain weaves his or her way under the arms of the other children in the chain to form a tangle.
- Without breaking the chain the children need to find a way to untangle themselves.

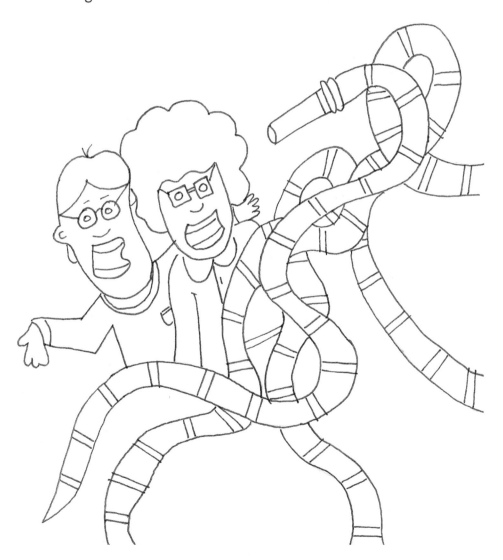

This exercise helps children to learn to work together and encourages problem-solving. Even if a problem is difficult to solve, by trying different ways you usually come to a solution in the end.

The beautiful hag

In the first picture below some people see an old hag while others see a young lady. The second picture can be seen as a vase or two faces looking at each other. Which do you see when you first look at the pictures? Tick or circle the boxes below:

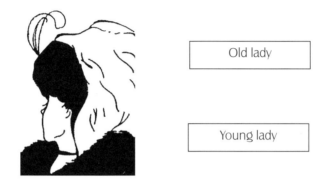

Old lady

Young lady

My Wife and My Mother in Law (1915). By W.E. Hill

Two faces

Vase

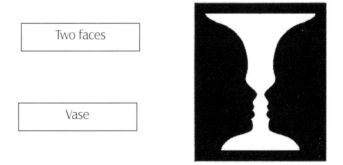

The Rubin Vase (1915). By E. Rubin

As you can see from these pictures there is often more than one way of looking at things. There are no right or wrong answers but the way we think about things does affect how we feel about them. For example, if you see an old hag in the first picture you may feel afraid and look away from the picture. However, if you see the beautiful lady you may feel happy and wish to meet her. In the second picture some children say they see two angry people and feel upset. Others say they are two lovers staring into each other's eyes. Find out what others in your group feel about the pictures.

Are you a Pollyanna?

Because everyone is different, people often have quite different thoughts about things. Some people always seem to see the good or positive things in everything and everybody while others only seem to see the bad or negative things in life. This is sometimes described as seeing a glass as half full or half empty.

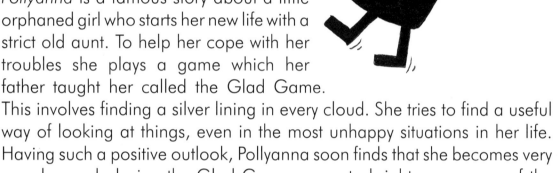

Pollyanna is a famous story about a little orphaned girl who starts her new life with a strict old aunt. To help her cope with her troubles she plays a game which her father taught her called the Glad Game. This involves finding a silver lining in every cloud. She tries to find a useful way of looking at things, even in the most unhappy situations in her life. Having such a positive outlook, Pollyanna soon finds that she becomes very popular, and playing the Glad Game seems to brighten up some of the unhappy characters she meets in the community she lives in.

Although trying to be positive is not always useful, you may find playing the Glad Game helps you to explore different ways of thinking about things, especially if you are feeling really stuck and unhappy. In the boxes below write the names of anyone you know who tends to think really negatively about everything, or like Pollyanna anyone you know who always seems to look on the bright or positive side of life.

Positive thinkers

Negative thinkers

The gloomies

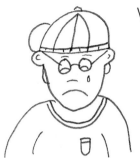

With gloomy thinking we focus only on negative things that happen. We notice all the things that go wrong. Anything positive tends to get overlooked, disbelieved or thought of as unimportant. It is as though we are wearing a 'gloomy thinking cap' or that we see everything through negative glasses. See the examples below:

You are asked to go to a party with someone you really like.
You think, 'They probably couldn't find anyone else to go with. That's why they're asking me.'

Harry did well in his maths test.
He thinks, 'Oh well, it was an easy test. If it was harder I would be sure to fail.'

A friend tells Katie: 'Your hair looks lovely today.'
'She's only saying that because she wants me to help her. She thinks I look ugly really.'

The gloomy thinking cap challenge

A volunteer from the group puts on the 'gloomy thinking cap'. While they are wearing the cap they can only see the negative or gloomy side of things. They see the worst in the world, themselves and everybody. The challenge is for other group members to try and make the person wearing the 'gloomy thinking cap' be cheerful and laugh or say something positive like Pollyanna. Each person in the group challenges the cap wearer with one question, a joke, or funny face. If the cap wearer laughs, smiles or says something positive, he or she has lost the challenge and someone else wears the 'gloomy thinking cap'.

Downward diggers

To understand what is upsetting you about a worry or problem make some cool connections by using a 'downward digger' question. For example:

What is the worst thing about that?

Or

What is the worst thing that could happen?

It may seem simple, but with a little practice and the help of a downward digger question it is possible to dig right to the heart of a problem or worry and see why it upsets you so much. Knowing what is at the bottom of your worry can be a big step to overcoming your problem or understanding other people's. See the examples below and then make up a problem and have a go with a friend. Show your downward digger to the group.

Downward digger 1

My problem is that I am scared to talk out in class
What is the worst thing that could happen if you had to talk in class?
I will make mistakes and stumble over the words
And if that were true what would be the worst thing about that?
Other kids will laugh at me
And if other kids laugh at you what would be the worst thing about that?
I will get really embarrassed and go very red
What's the worst thing about going red?
I will look stupid
What's the worst thing about looking stupid?
Kids in the class will think I'm stupid
What's so bad about that?
I'll think I'm stupid

Downward digger 2

My problem is maths in school
What's the worst thing about maths?
I keep getting told off by my teacher
What's the worst thing about that?
He gets really mad and shouts
What's the worst thing that could happen?
I could get a detention
What's the worst thing about that?
My parents might find out
What's the worst thing about that?
They will get really upset with me
What's the worst thing that could happen?
They will think I'm a bad kid
What's the worst thing about that?
They will stop caring about me
What's the worst thing that could happen?
I'll know I'm a bad kid
And if you are a bad kid what's the worst thing about that?
No-one will like me and I'll end up sad and lonely forever

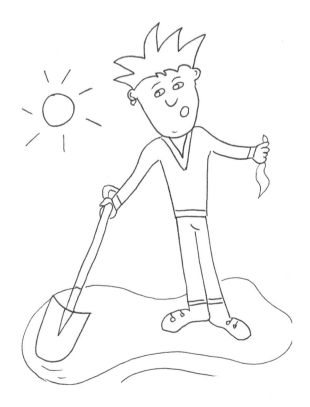

My downward digger

Choose a puppet to work with. Make up something that your puppet may be frightened or upset about and then write it in the box below. Make sure you only write one worry – rather than a complete story! For example, 'My puppet is worried that he has no friends', or 'My puppet is upset because he thinks he looks weird', etc.

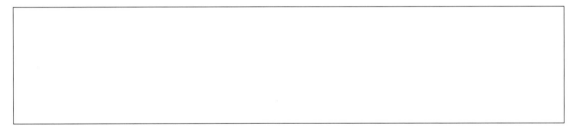

After the downward digger, what thoughts were at the heart of your puppet's fears? Write some of the things that were most upsetting for the puppet in the box below. For example, your puppet may feel deep down that it is totally bad, stupid, ugly, useless, lonely, etc. Use the puppet's own words to describe his or her feelings.

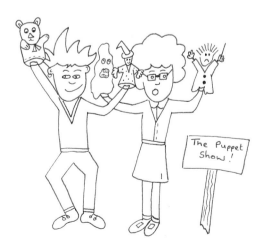

Helping hands

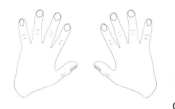 As you can see from the downward digger exercise it is useful to become more aware of the thoughts which are making you feel gloomy or afraid. With this information you have more choice as to what to do next. Once you have caught yourself wearing a 'gloomy thinking cap' and have worked out your 'downward digger' thoughts it is time to take action. It is not useful to let yourself spend too much time thinking over and over about your upset or worrying thoughts. Below are two actions you can take.

1.   Talk to someone you trust about how you feel. Perhaps they could give you a 'helping hand'. This could be your parents, a family member, teacher, or friend. Write the names of people who can support you in the box below:

2.   You can also help yourself by doing something you enjoy. Sometimes when people feel upset they don't feel like doing anything at all. The truth is that if you don't do anything you are likely to feel more upset and very stuck. Get out and do an activity you enjoy and you will feel better much more quickly. In the box below write some activities you enjoy doing and share them with the group. This could be football or swimming, drawing, painting, dancing, etc.

If you have time you may want to experiment with the above idea. Try imagining yourself doing one of the activities you have written in the box and see how it makes you feel.

Wise worriers

Often people have worrying thoughts which go round and round in their heads. The trouble is that the more worrying thoughts they have the more worried and upset they feel. These thoughts usually start with 'what if' questions which often never get answered.

As well as talking to someone you trust and doing something you enjoy (see page 140) a third way of helping yourself with worrying thoughts is to practise answering your 'what if' questions with 'then I can do' answers. Practise this. It can calm you down and help you cope. You may also find this useful in helping your friends sort their worries out. Complete some of the questions on the next page. Compare your answers with the rest of the group. In the blank row at the bottom see if you can make up a 'what if' question and a 'then I can do' answer of your own.

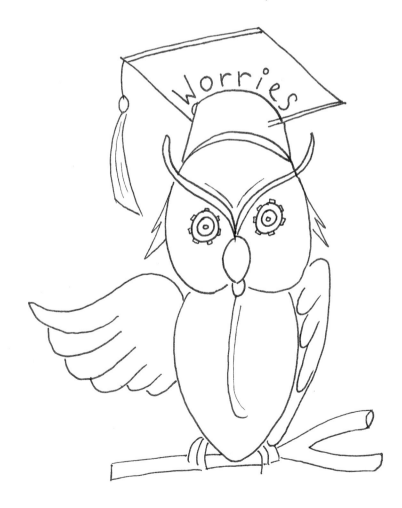

COOL CONNECTIONS WITH CBT

'What if' question	'Then I can do' answer
Example: What if I can't answer the questions in English today?	Then I can ask for help from my friend. Making mistakes is a good way to learn new things.
Example: What if I fall in the river while we are on holiday?	I can be prepared by wearing a life jacket. I will tell my friends I can't swim before we leave. I will shout and scream for help. Someone will save me. Lots of people are going to be around.
What if I make a mistake in my school work?	
What if I get bullied at school? The bullies are so big.	
What if I cry in public? It will be so embarrassing.	
What if I get a serious illness?	
What if someone I care about gets attacked or dies?	

Copyright © Laurie Seiler 2008

Home Activity 6: Eavesdropping

Listen to your friends, family and teachers this week and see if you can spot them talking as though they are wearing a 'gloomy thinking cap' or speaking like Pollyanna in her Glad Game (see page 133–134). Briefly write who and what they have said in the boxes below.

Child = C Adult = A	Pollyanna = P Gloomy = G	What did they say?
Example: A	G	No-one ever hands in their homework
Example: C	P	I learn something new every day

SESSION 7: Exploring Thoughts

Aims and objectives

- Learn how to explore alternative ways of looking at your difficulties.
- Become 'scientific' in your approach to problem-solving by looking for evidence and facts rather than myth and speculation.
- Observe how 'green light thoughts' can improve how you feel.

Materials

Chairs, pencils.

Agenda and tips for running the session

Exercises in bold in the left-hand column should be included in both long and short sessions. Other exercises are optional and can be included in groups where there is more time. Many fun activities/games are included as optional. Despite sometimes being short of time it is important not to cut all the 'fun' out of the programme or you will lose the children's enthusiasm.

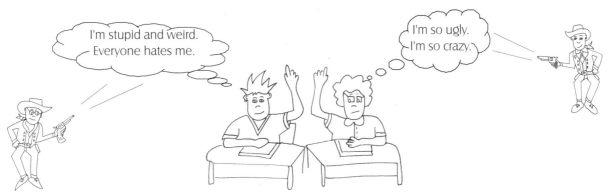

Short session

EXERCISE	COMMENTS
Feedback	Welcome the children and share agenda for session with group. Obtain brief feedback from children's week.
Review Home Activity 6	Children can briefly discuss their findings following the eavesdropping exercise. What did they notice? Facilitators collect home activities to explore in more detail after the session and return the following week or at the end of the programme.
Thought–feeling cool connections	Encourage children to make the connection between their thoughts and the way they feel. Children can be asked to share one answer with the rest of the group. If children make different connections from the rest of the group this can be discussed openly in a non-judgemental way.
Traffic light thinking	Makes a link between different types of thinking and a traffic light system. Children do not need to focus too much on amber thoughts (observational-type thoughts). However, they have been included to help prevent children exploring their thoughts in 'black and white' or inflexible ways. For example, green thoughts are 'good' and red thoughts are 'bad'.
Red light, green light	Children write red light and green light thoughts in the thought bubbles. There are no right or wrong answers. Children share the contents of one of their thought bubbles with the group.
Red, amber, green	It is important that there is a noticeable difference between the way the swimmer behaves when the children are cheering and saying green light thoughts and when they are booing and/or saying red light thoughts. It can be useful to compare this exercise with how children often say red light thoughts to themselves, e.g. 'You idiot' when making a mistake. How useful are the things we say to ourselves?

Changing those red light thoughts	Children are encouraged to share with the group an example of how they have changed a red light thought to a more useful green light thought.
Traffic lights thought contest	Read the example in the thought bubbles to the group. Children could use drawings, models or puppets. Children show their scenes to the group. The participants are asked how it felt to play the different parts. The group can be asked whether the red or green light thoughts were the most powerful, useful, calming, etc. This can be compared with how much or little the children listen to their own red light thoughts.
Example: Red light thought challenge	Read through the example. The children may wish to read; however, this can take more time. Ask the children to compare this exercise with the traffic lights thought contest exercise.
Red light thought challenge	Red light thoughts described about other children are often thoughts which children have about themselves. However, this is not always the case. This exercise can sometimes make children feel low, especially if they struggle to find evidence against their red light thoughts. Other group members can be encouraged to offer support and/or help with this. See Notes on page 146.
Home Activity 7a: Thinking quiz	Children practise identifying unhelpful and helpful thoughts.
Home Activity 7b: Red light thought challenge	Children practise the exercise on page 155. The exercise aims to help children explore different ways of thinking. Finding more useful ways of thinking should help improve the children's mood and reduce anxious, angry or helpless feelings.

Long session

Include 'Red, amber, green' on page 151. This exercise can be changed to suit the group (e.g. the swimmer could be a climber or a runner). More time can be spent on the 'Traffic lights thought contest' exercise (page 153). Children can be invited to share examples of red light or green light thoughts that have been said to them by teachers, friends, etc. Clips from magazines could be cut out and the children can connect red light or green light thoughts to the pictures and share these with the group.

Notes

The exercises in this session aim to help children further explore alternative ways of thinking about things. We have a tendency to believe the red light thoughts that we say to ourselves and act as though they are true. Although in some cases they may be true, generally the red light or negative things we say to ourselves are not 100 per cent fact. By catching our red light thoughts (pages 105 and 106) we begin to reflect upon them and explore evidence of their accuracy. Research suggests that the more evidence (or green light thoughts) we find to contradict our negative or red light thoughts the better we feel. The trouble with red light thoughts is that, although they are often intended to help motivate or protect us, the outcome is usually that they end up making us feel unhappy, angry, worried, more self-critical and often very stuck. This then causes a vicious circle (red light thoughts = unhappy feelings = more red light thoughts). The exercise on page 155 is difficult and will take frequent practice.

Thought–feeling cool connections

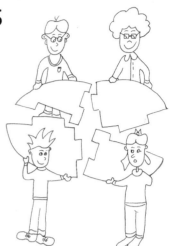

In the last session we made cool connections about different ways of thinking. Some people think in positive ways, like Pollyanna with her 'Glad Game', while others seem to wear their 'gloomy thinking caps' and see things in negative ways that seem to keep them stuck. Most people have a mixture of both types of thinking in different situations. However, when we get upset, angry or worried, it is common for us to put on our 'gloomy thinking caps' and assume the worst about ourselves, everything and everyone. In this session we are going to make some more connections about our thinking. In the following exercise be cool and connect the following thoughts in the left-hand column with the feelings in the right-hand column.

Thoughts	Feelings
I've got no friends because I'm a horrible person.	Happy
I can do it if I try.	Sad
I've coped with harder things than this before. The big wheel could be fun.	Angry
I want to hit all the other children at school.	Worried
I can always ask for help if I can't do it.	Confident
I just can't cope. It's just too hard.	Excited

Which do you think are the 'glad' thoughts, as in Pollyanna's 'Glad Game', and how can you tell?

Traffic light thinking

We have already learned cool connections about the way our thoughts affect our feelings. Like scientists we are now going to explore the thoughts which connect with our upset, angry or worried feelings. To do this we will begin by challenging the thoughts which keep us stuck. To do this you may find it helpful to imagine your thoughts as the colours of a traffic light system.

Red light thoughts usually make us feel more upset, worried or angry. They seem to hold us back and keep us feeling helpless and stuck in a vicious cycle. These thoughts often make us more aware of danger and the worst thing that can happen to us or other people.

Green light thoughts are soothing or calming thoughts which make us feel better about ourselves and/or our situation. Green light thoughts are useful and can help us cope better. These are 'doing' thoughts which help us take purposeful action towards achieving our goals.

Amber light thoughts are noticing or observational thoughts. There is no positive or negative value placed upon them. They are just thoughts that pop into our minds and then float off again, like a gentle breeze on a summer's day. Although amber thoughts may help us become more aware of things around us they are less important in making the cool connections needed to help us explore the thoughts which cause us to feel so upset, worried or angry. If all thoughts were amber we might well feel peaceful but we might also never get anything done. See the two examples of traffic light thinking on the next page.

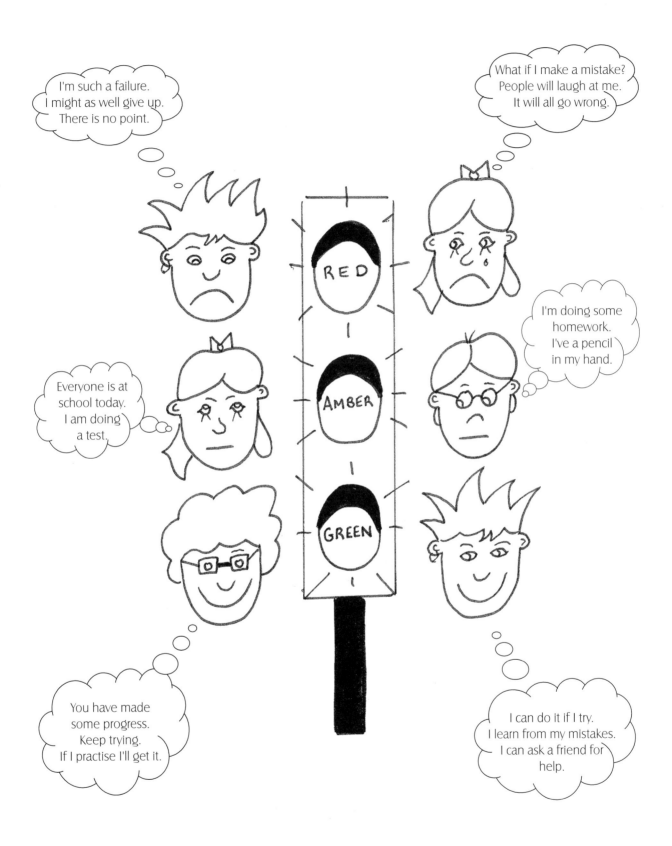

Red light, green light

Write a green light thought and a red light thought for each of the pictures with empty thought bubbles.

Example

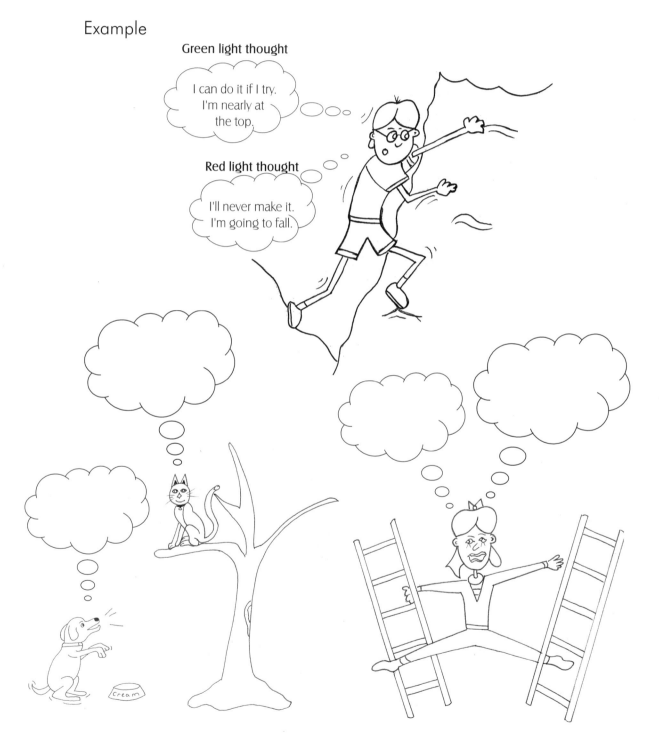

Green light thought

I can do it if I try. I'm nearly at the top.

Red light thought

I'll never make it. I'm going to fall.

Red, amber, green

The aim of this exercise is to experiment and see the effect our thinking can have on our actions. A volunteer from the group lies tummy downwards across a chair or a bench. He or she is asked to imagine that they are swimming in a race at the swimming pool. As the child pretends to swim the rest of the group are encouraged to shout red light thoughts such as 'You'll never make it' or 'You're so slow', etc. Following this exercise the group members experiment by cheering and offering the swimmer green light thoughts such as 'You are doing great' or 'Come on, you are nearly there'.

What effect did the red light thoughts have on the swimmer?

_____

_____

What effect did the green light thoughts have on the swimmer?

_____

_____

Give an example of an amber thought the swimmer may have had.

_____

_____

Changing those red light thoughts

Choose two of the red light thoughts below and see if you can change them into green light thoughts.

Example

RED LIGHT THOUGHT

'Everyone hates me because I'm so ugly. My hair is disgusting, my nose is too long and my legs are like bean poles.'

GREEN LIGHT THOUGHT

'I know that I feel like I'm ugly sometimes but it doesn't mean that I really am. No-one has actually said I'm ugly. Anyway I am good at sports, English and music. My friends say I'm good company.'

Red light thoughts

1. I'll never be able to climb the mountain. It's just too high.

2. There is no point in trying to join the sports team. They will only pick the good players and I never do well at anything.

3. Donald and Daffy Duck keep picking on me. I'm never going back to that stupid duck school. It's 're-duckulous'. Everyone thinks I'm totally quackers.

4. I'm feeling dizzy and sick again. Oh no, help, help, I'm probably going to die. No, please, not here in school. The other kids will see. I need my Mum NOW. I feel dizzy. It's getting worse. Don't let me pass out and die. Arrrrrrh!

GREEN LIGHT THOUGHT

– –

GREEN LIGHT THOUGHT

– –

Traffic lights thought contest

Make a group of three with your friends and act out the following scene:

- Person 1. Act or draw a situation or goal that may be difficult for you to achieve. For example, climbing a mountain, reading out loud, or confronting a bully.

- Person 2. Become Person 1's red light thoughts. Try and stop Person 1 achieving the goal by saying negative thoughts to him or her. You may argue with Person 3 if you wish.

- Person 3. You have become Person 1's green light thoughts. Try and help Person 1 achieve their goal by saying useful or calming thoughts to him or her. You may argue with Person 2 if you wish.

- Show your scene to the rest of the group. Discuss what effect the red light and green light thoughts might have on Person 1's feelings and actions.

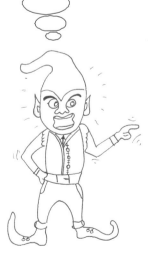

RED LIGHT THOUGHTS

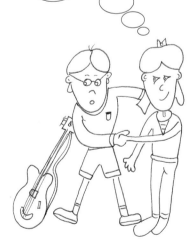

GREEN LIGHT THOUGHTS

Example: Red light thought challenge

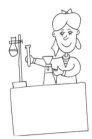

Like a scientist looking for evidence we are going to learn cool ways to test out thoughts which make us feel upset or worried. In the following exercise think of a red light thought that a friend might have about themselves. For example, 'I'm stupid' or 'No-one likes me'. Having identified a thought see if you can explore the evidence as shown in the example below.

This is a red light thought a friend might have about themselves:

I am totally boring

How much on a score 0–10 do you think your friend believes their red light thought?

Evidence which says my friend's red light thought is 'completely' true	Evidence which says my friend's red light thought is not 'completely' true
• His friends said that they could not go out with him at the weekend. • He had to stay at home on his own. • He does not like football like other kids. • Some kids at school call him a boffin. • He sometimes thinks that he does not fit in at school.	• No-one has actually said that he is boring – only himself. • If he was boring he would have no friends. Actually he has got quite a few. • Lots of kids don't like football. It does not mean he is boring. Anyway, he does like snooker and fishing. • There are lots of other reasons why his friends may not be able to see him at the weekend – they may be grounded. • Everyone thinks they don't fit in sometimes. It does not always mean it is true.

How much on a score 0–10 do you think your friend believes their red light thought now?

Red light thought challenge

Now it is your turn. Choose a red light thought that you or someone else might have about themselves. Like a scientist try and explore some green light thoughts or more useful, calming thoughts to challenge the red light thought. Don't forget to rate the thought both before and after challenging it. This is difficult – good luck!

Red light thought you or a friend might have about themselves:

How much on a score 0–10 do you think your friend believes their red light thought?

Evidence which says the red light thought is 'completely' true	Evidence which says the red light thought is not 'completely' true

How much on a score of 0–10 do you or your friend believe their red light thought now?

Home Activity 7a: Thinking quiz

Tick the boxes on the right to show green light thoughts or red light thoughts	Green light thoughts	Red light thoughts
I'm just totally stupid.		
They only want me to play because they can't find anyone else.		
I'm good at a lot of things but if I'm not the best I always give up.		
They will all laugh at me if I go out dressed in these clothes.		
I can do it if I try.		
I'm so ugly.		
Someone will help me out if I get stuck.		
I won't bother going fishing on Saturday. I never catch anything anyway.		
I'm trying really hard with my homework because if I don't my mum will shout at me.		
If I am upset or worried I can tell people how I feel.		
I'm the best guitarist in the world.		
If I think about car crashes I might be in one.		
I hate school and everything about it.		
Some people like me and some don't – that's the way of the world.		
My worries make me feel like I'm going crazy.		
Just because I think there is a monster under my bed does not mean that there is.		
I'm totally rubbish at everything.		
I may not have done well this time but I really enjoyed taking part.		

Home Activity 7b: Red light thought challenge

Next time you feel upset or worried check out one of your red light thoughts. Like a scientist try and explore evidence for and against the red light thought. After you have identified and rated your thought between 0–10 write down all the reasons why your red light thought is true. Having done this, see if you can find any evidence to say that the thought is not true. This is difficult and can take a lot of practice. Don't give up – and good luck.

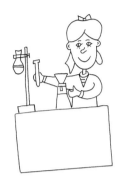

Red light thought you have about yourself (I'm stupid, ugly, boring, etc.):

How much on a score 0–10 do you think you believe your red light thought?

Evidence which says my red light thought is 'completely' true	Evidence which says my red light thought is not 'completely' true

How much on a score of 0–10 do you believe your red light thought now?

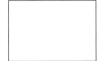

SESSION 8: Goal Setting

Aims and objectives

- Make a six-point plan for goal setting.
- Encourage the group to work together and support each other through difficulties.
- Help the group to be clear and specific about their difficulties.
- Learn from watching others goal setting.

Materials

Chairs, pencils, selection of hoops.

Agenda and tips for running the session

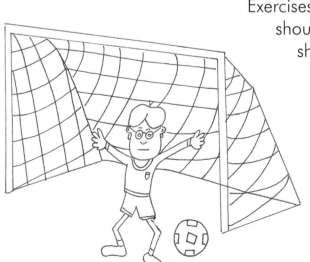

Exercises in bold in the left-hand column should be included in both long and short sessions. Other exercises are optional and can be included in groups where there is more time. Many fun activities/games are included as optional. Despite sometimes being short of time it is important not to cut all the 'fun' out of the programme or you will lose the children's enthusiasm.

Short session

EXERCISE	COMMENTS
Feedback	Welcome the children and share agenda for session with group. Obtain brief feedback from children's week.
Review Home Activities 7a and 7b	Children can briefly discuss Home Activities 7a and 7b. Facilitators collect home activities to explore in more detail after the session and return the following week or at the end of the programme.
Murder mystery	Children are encouraged to make connections between the skills required to find the murderer (observing others, listening, etc.) and the skills required for problem-solving and/or goal setting. Questions can be asked; for example, 'What did you need to do to catch the murderer?' 'How did you find out?' 'Which of your five senses did you use?' 'What happened if your guess was incorrect?'
IT solutions	This exercise is similar to the above. Some older groups of children may prefer this activity.
As clear as mud	Encourage the children to read the different parts on page 164. Ask different children to share their answers with the group.
Hoola hoola	You will need a clear space to complete this exercise (sports hall or playground). The children find a partner. They are then given a hoop and asked to complete the exercise stages A–F before feeding back to the group. It is important that children work together, generating ideas and exploring possible consequences in sections A–D before putting their ideas into practice. Time is given for the children to practise and change their plan before the race commences. Following the race children are asked to report back to the group about their outcomes. If facilitators prefer, a balloon or ball could be used instead of a hoop.

Home Activity 8a: **Superstars**	It is useful to observe how other people cope with problems. Children learn a lot about coping with problems by observing others with good coping skills.
Home Activity 8b: **Goal Setting**	Children practise the exercise they have learned on pages 166–167.

Long session

Include 'IT solutions'. 'Superstars' can be incorporated into the main session rather than as a home activity exercise. Either in addition or as an alternative, a secret treasure (pieces of fruit or small sweets) can be hidden round the room while the children have their eyes closed. The children are then given a limited time to find the treasure and return to their seats. The children are asked what they did in order to find the treasure (listening, trying one place then another, watching others, etc.). The 'Hoola hoola' game can be extended either by providing every child with their own hoop or by dividing the group in half and having one hoop per team. If you have the time, short stories or video/DVD clips demonstrating good problem-solving or goal-setting skills can also be included. Some discussion about family members, friends or famous people who are good at solving problems or setting goals, and why, may also be helpful.

Murder mystery

- One child volunteers to be a detective. He or she is asked to leave the room while the other group members decide who will act as a murderer.

- The murderer kills his victims by winking at them. Should group members be winked at by the murderer they should pretend to die 'loudly' and lie on the floor as if they were dead.

- When all members of the group are ready the detective is invited back into the room. He or she must use detective skills to identify who the murderer is.

- When the murderer is found, the game is ended. You may wish to swap roles and play again.

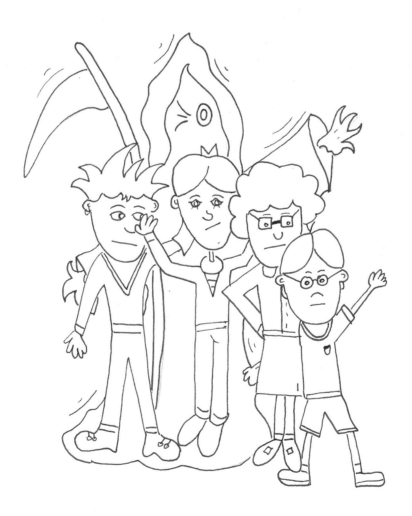

IT solutions

Many of you have already become very good at finding solutions to difficult situations. In the computer screen below write your favourite computer game. In the outer boxes write the different things you had to do to reach your goal and become skilled at this game. For example, how did you defeat the dragon? Climb the waterfall? Get through to the next level? You might find it helpful to think of the tips you would give a friend playing the game for the first time.

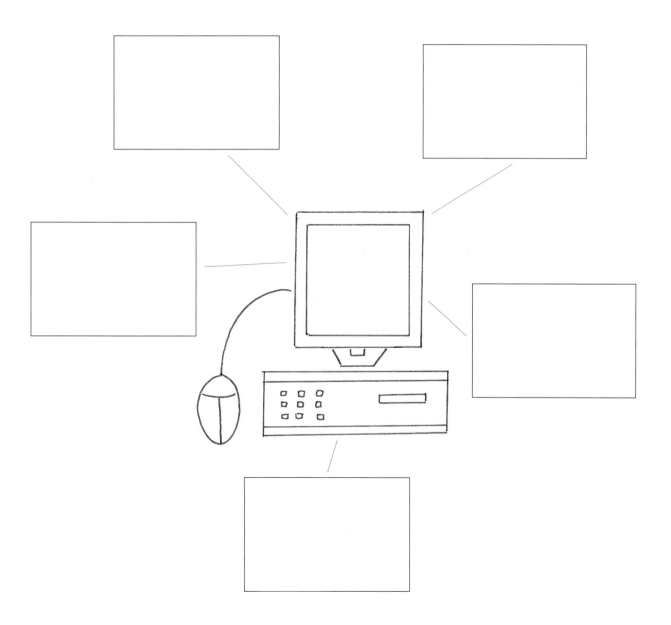

As clear as mud

Many children find it difficult to describe their problems and their goals. They often know something is wrong and they are unhappy but can't explain why. The first cool connection you need to make towards reaching your goal is becoming clear about exactly what is bothering you and where you want to get to. To do this you will need to learn how to be specific and clear like a mountain stream rather than too big and unclear like a muddy river. Make cool connections about which statements are muddy and which are clear from the following examples.

JACK: I hate school and I'm not going back to that dump.

PARENT: What is it about school that is troubling you?

JACK: Everything. I hate everything about school. It's just horrid.

PARENT: Has something happened you are not telling me about?

JACK: No, I just hate school and I'm never ever going back there.

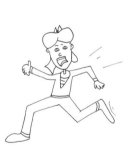

LAUREN: I hate school and I'm not going back to that dump.

PARENT: What is it about school that is troubling you?

LAUREN: I hate break times the most.

PARENT: What is it that is so bad about break times?

LAUREN: Other kids keep calling me a boffin 'cause I'm good at maths and stuff.

PARENT: And what is so bad about being called a boffin?

LAUREN: It makes me feel I'm different like a weird kid or something.

Which child above has most clearly described their problems at school, Jack or Lauren?

If you were a teacher or parent do you think it would be easier to help Jack or Lauren? Give your reason below:

If you were a teacher or parent trying to help Jack how would you feel?

From the following problems highlight which are specific and clear and which are too big and muddy.

I'm sure I've got something really wrong with me.

I'm worried because I had a sick feeling in my stomach during games.

I get bullied all the time by everyone at school.

Harry was hitting me again during first break.

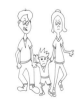

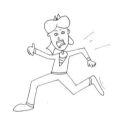

I'm just totally ugly and everyone hates me.

I don't like my hair style. It makes me look different from other kids.

My parents got cross with me this morning because I was late for school again.

Everybody hates me in my family.

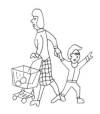

Shopping is so boring I never get anything I want.

I need some of those big gobstopper sweets up there, Mum.

Hoola hoola

Your mission is to solve the following problem by using the A–F goal-setting plan. With the help of a partner take a hoop and try to get it from one side of the room to the other without touching the hoop with your hands or feet. Think about what you are going to do, and complete the answers to A–D, before you get going with your hoop.

(A) What is your goal?

_ _

_ _

(B) What could you do to make your goal happen? (ideas)

1. _

2. _

3. _

(C) What could stop you reaching your goal? (consequences)

1. _

2. _

3. _

(D) Which of your ideas do you think will work best?

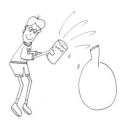

_ _

_ _

(E) Experiment and try out your plan with your partner.

(F) What happened? Did it work?

Positive outcomes	Things to improve

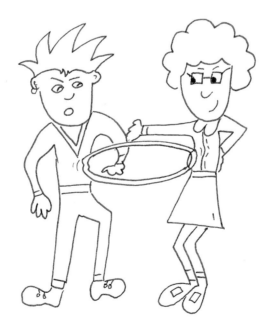

Home Activity 8a: Superstars

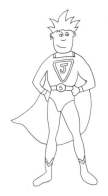

Sometimes when people get stressed it can be difficult to think of good goal-setting ideas. On these occasions people can feel very stuck. The more stuck they feel the more stressed they get, like a vicious circle. When you get stuck like this you can get some good ideas for goal setting by thinking about how other people might cope if they were in the same situation. Think of a person you look up to or who you think copes well in stressful or difficult situations. This could be a superstar from the TV, a cartoon character, a family member, or even a friend. Complete the information below.

Describe a problem that you think would be very scary or stressful.

[ ]

Write a goal for making the problem better. (How would you like things to be?)

[ ]

Write the name of a person or superstar whom you believe would cope well with this situation. (The superstar does not have to be a real person.)

[ ]

How would your superstar cope with the scary or stressful situation? What would they do and how would they feel inside?

[ ]

Home Activity 8b: Goal setting

Your mission this week is to identify something in your life that is troubling you. Use the A–F goal-setting plan to help you achieve your goal.

(A) What is your goal?

_ _

_ _

_ _

(B) What could you do to make your goal happen? (ideas)

1. _

2. _

3. _

(C) What could stop you reaching your goal? (consequences)

1. _

2. _

3. _

(D) Which of your ideas do you think will work best?

_ _

_ _

_ _

(E) Experiment and try out your plan with your partner.

(F) What happened? Did it work?

Positive outcomes	Things to improve

SESSION 9: Panic Cycles and Safety Seeking Actions

Aims and objectives

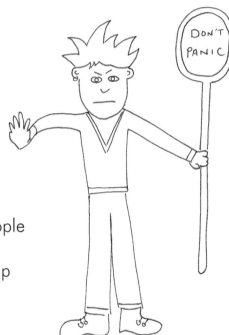

- Learn cool connections about how everyone is different and worries about different things.

- See how some of your thoughts and feelings can keep you feeling stuck.

- Find out the different things that people do to protect themselves from their worries and how these can often help feed the problem.

Materials

Chairs, pencils.

Agenda and tips for running the session

Exercises in bold in the left-hand column should be included in both long and short sessions. Other exercises are optional and can be included in groups where there is more time. Many fun activities/games are included as optional. Despite sometimes being short of time it is important not to cut all the 'fun' out of the programme or you will lose the children's enthusiasm.

Short session

EXERCISE	COMMENTS
Feedback	Welcome the children and share agenda for session with group. Obtain brief feedback from children's week.
Review Home Activities 8a and 8b	Children can briefly share one or both home activities. Facilitators collect home activities to explore in more detail after the session and return the following week or at the end of the programme.
The swamp monster	You need a lot of space. Perhaps start the session with this game in a hall or playground. Encourage the children to make the connection between having worries and/or upset feelings and how these can make you feel very helpless and stuck.
Everyone is different	Some children enjoy reading and can be made to feel more involved. However, this can slow the session down. Children share one or two of the things which they have circled as important to them with the group.
Don't panic!	This exercise helps children to see the links between their thoughts and feelings. Children should be encouraged to notice how worrying thoughts increase physical sensations, forming a vicious cycle.
Put safety first!	Read the story about the children on the train and Jack and his vampires. Many of the children often seem perplexed initially but eventually most will get the idea. The children can answer the questions on page 180, either alone or with a partner, and feed back to the group. If you have limited time read a few of the examples on pages 180–181 and ask the children to feed back verbally the safety seeking actions. Children can then be divided into small groups, given a character from the exercise (Lauren, Katie, Jack or Harry), and asked to either draw, act or identify what they could do differently to overcome their fear.

My safety seeking actions	If children cannot name something they are afraid of they can make something up or choose something they know someone else is afraid of.
Home Activity 9a: Hidden worries	Children are encouraged to observe their avoidant behaviours.
Home Activity 9b: What do I do?	This helps children develop an understanding of their own safety seeking actions. Children are encouraged to look at how these actions can help or hinder them from coping with their fears.

Long session

Include 'The swamp monster' game. Show an example of safety seeking actions from a story or video/DVD clip. The classic Disney cartoon *Dumbo* is an excellent example. In the film the little elephant 'Dumbo' believes that the only reason he can fly is because he is holding the feather of a bird. It is not until he drops the feather by accident that he suddenly realizes that he can fly without it. In the exercises on pages 180–181 children can be given more time to choose the characters they would like to act for themselves.

Note

We have found it useful to suggest that children indicate with a large cross if any of the characters on pages 180–181 remind them of themselves. Although most people can identify with all the characters at some point in their lives, children identifying themselves as very similar to the characters (Lauren, Katie, Jack and Harry) on a frequent basis will require further investigation. (These are similar symptoms to those of anxiety disorders such as social phobia, obsessive compulsive disorder, or panic attacks).

The swamp monster

A dangerous and dirty swamp monster has escaped from the depths of a muddy swamp in the land of Piggiwinkles.

If he touches you with his magical muddy fingers you will automatically be stuck like the pig below in a muddy swamp. The only way to be freed from the swamp monster's swampy spell is for another member of your group to crawl through your legs.

If everyone gets swamped by the swamp monster then his powers get stronger and he is the winner.

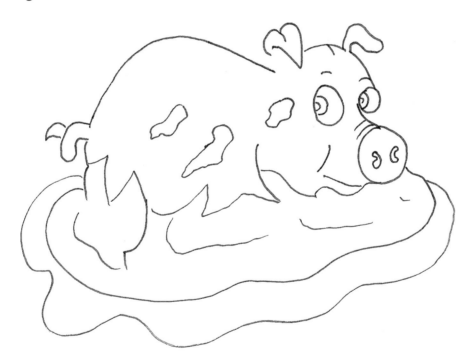

This session helps to show us that:
- sometimes our problems and worries can make us feel very stuck
- sometimes the things we do to help us escape can make us even more stuck
- running away from our fears can make us feel more stuck
- it is good to ask someone to help even if the problem seems too big.

Everyone is different

Everyone is different and will worry about different things. This depends on their values and the things which are important to them. We usually get these values from the experiences we have had in our lives or sometimes from our families. If someone in your family has a strong view about something you may well share their opinion.

Lauren's mother often tells her that it is wrong to drop litter. Lauren also thinks this is a 'bad' thing to do. On the other hand, Jack's mother often throws rubbish out of her car window as she is driving along. Not surprisingly Jack often drops litter in the street and does not seem bothered about the mess at all. Listed below are some of the things which are important to some children. Circle the things below that are important to you.

Being liked by other kids	Being good at sports	Being helpful and kind
Being thin	Being clever at my work in school	Being perfect and not making any mistakes
Being tough and hard	Being different from everyone else	Being happy at home and with family
Being caring to animals	Being good at making or fixing things	Being attractive to others

The things you have circled above are very important to you. Because of this you are likely to worry about them. Should something go wrong or you feel you are failing in one of these areas you are likely to feel very upset. This is sometimes called a trigger. Because we are all different we all have different triggers for our worries.

Take Fido the dog on the left, for example. If someone tried to take his bone he would become very upset and worried. Felix, on the other hand, is not interested in bones so she wouldn't care who has the bone. However, just you stay away from her cream!

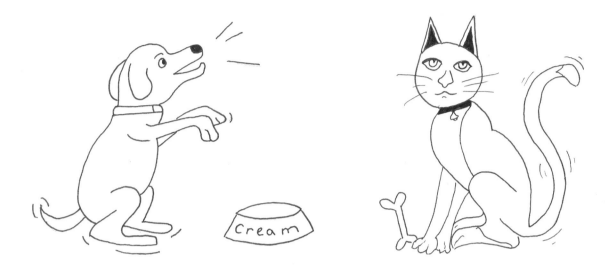

Don't panic!

When people worry it is always about things in the future and what is *going* to happen rather than what has happened in the past. It can be very easy to get caught up in a vicious cycle which can make you feel more and more scared and stuck. This cycle is sometimes called the cycle of panic. See the examples of Jack and Katie below:

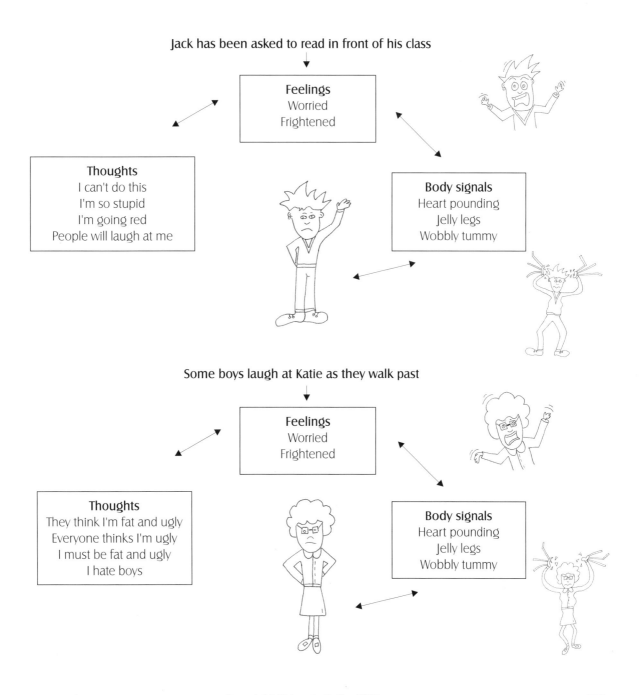

Jack has been asked to read in front of his class

Feelings
Worried
Frightened

Thoughts
I can't do this
I'm so stupid
I'm going red
People will laugh at me

Body signals
Heart pounding
Jelly legs
Wobbly tummy

Some boys laugh at Katie as they walk past

Feelings
Worried
Frightened

Thoughts
They think I'm fat and ugly
Everyone thinks I'm ugly
I must be fat and ugly
I hate boys

Body signals
Heart pounding
Jelly legs
Wobbly tummy

Jack and Katie were bullied during break time. They fear it could happen again this break time.

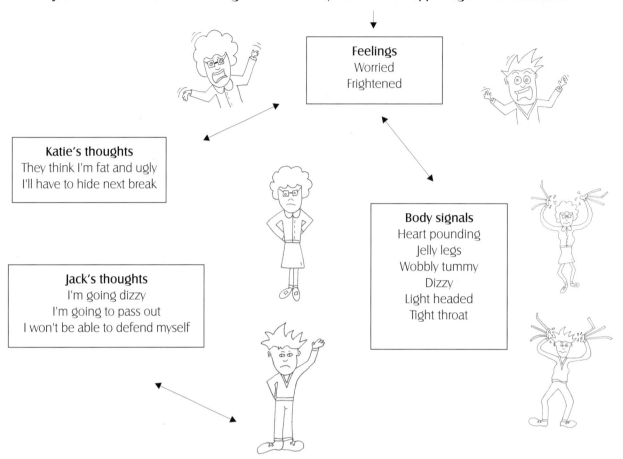

Feelings
Worried
Frightened

Katie's thoughts
They think I'm fat and ugly
I'll have to hide next break

Jack's thoughts
I'm going dizzy
I'm going to pass out
I won't be able to defend myself

Body signals
Heart pounding
Jelly legs
Wobbly tummy
Dizzy
Light headed
Tight throat

Make cool connections by noticing how in different situations both Katie and Jack's worries were different. This is because different things are important to them. Katie seems worried about her good looks and Jack about being physically harmed. Think of a time you have felt worried. In the boxes below see if you can map out your worry cycle:

What happened that made you worried? _ _ _ _ _ _ _ _ _ _ _ _ _ _ _ _ _ _ _

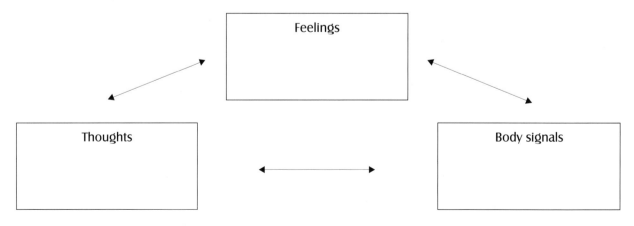

Feelings

Thoughts

Body signals

Put safety first!

Because worrying can be very uncomfortable and causes vicious cycles people often do things to try and break out. These are called safety seeking actions. The trouble is that safety seeking actions often trick you because they seem to help get rid of your worries for a while but then they come back again and can make you feel even more stuck and scared. The following short stories give examples of safety seeking actions.

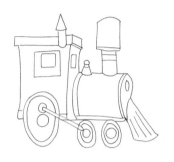

A small group of children are on a train throwing pieces of paper in the air. An older boy calls out, 'What are you doing?' They reply, 'Keeping elephants out of the train.' The older boy looks surprised and shouts back, 'But there are no elephants in this country and certainly not on this 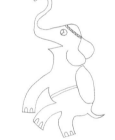 train.' 'Yes,' said the children playfully. 'Our strategy works really well doesn't it!'

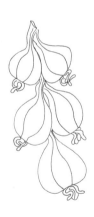

Jack invites his three friends – Harry, Katie and Lauren – to his house for a special party tea which he has cooked himself. When they arrive they notice lots of garlic hanging from the doorway and neatly placed across the windowsill in the kitchen. 'Strange,' they thought, but they didn't like to ask. 'Perhaps they are for the party?' Jack proudly presented the first course which was garlic bread. Very tasty too! For the main course Jack had made garlic chicken which arrived on a tray with rather odd tasting drinks in garlic-shaped glasses. Finally, for pudding his friends laughed when he produced a special type of garlic ice cream. Jack seemed puzzled as to why his guests were laughing, so eventually Lauren asked, 'What is it with all the garlic?' Jack was silent for a minute, then he said in a very serious tone, 'It's to keep the vampires away of course.' Harry, Katie and Lauren laughed again before Harry said, 'But there are no vampires.' 'Exactly,' said Jack, smiling to himself. 'The garlic has kept them away.'

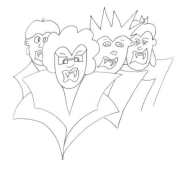

Why did Jack keep so much garlic in his house?

What safety seeking actions did Jack do to keep himself safe?

Do you think Jack's idea about keeping so much garlic is helping him overcome his fear of vampires? If so, how?

What would have to happen for Jack to find out the vampires do not exist? How would you advise him?

With a partner, make cool connections by seeing how many safety seeking actions you can detect from the characters below and circle each one. Choose one character and show (by acting, writing or drawing) what they could do differently to help them cope with or overcome their fear.

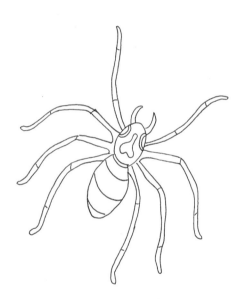

Lauren is scared of spiders. Each time she sees one she starts to feel panicky and runs away as fast as she can. Although she feels better when she gets away from the spider, she feels really silly next time she sees her friends. She spends a lot of time looking for spiders and won't go into a room if she so much as sees something that looks like a spider. She spends more time looking for spiders than doing her lessons.

Katie is worried about what people think of her so she spends hours practising what she says to people in her mirror at home just in case she says the wrong thing. Unless she has practised what to say she does not speak most of the time just in case she upsets someone.

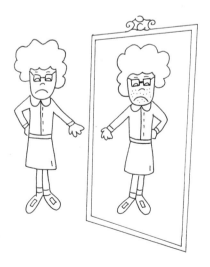

Jack is worried about catching germs so he washes his hands over and over again to prevent getting germs and being ill. If he doesn't wash his hands in a certain order he feels he must start washing them all over again. With all this washing his hands have become quite sore.

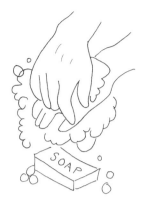

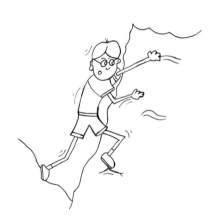

Harry's dad died of a heart attack. Sometimes when he gets panicky his chest gets tight and he thinks he will pass out and have a heart attack too. Even though the doctor has said there is nothing wrong with him he always holds on to something to stop himself falling if he feels worried. Just in case!

Jack does not like school because he keeps getting into trouble. He gets really panicky just thinking about school. He tells his mum that he has got a headache or feels sick. She lets him stay at home because she is so worried. Jack gets bored at home but he won't go back, just in case the horrid feelings of worry come back too.

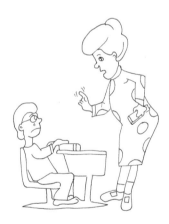

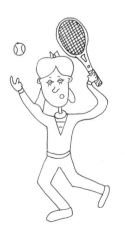

Lauren plays tennis in a top club. She is very good and has never lost a match. The first time she played in a tennis match someone told her that she would play well if she spins her racket ten times before each service. She is fed up with doing this now but is worried that if she stops she will lose the match.

My safety seeking actions

Name something that you are afraid of (For example, spiders, heights, parents arguing, blushing in public, etc.)

What things do you do to avoid facing your fear or stop it happening?
(For example, washing your hands to avoid germs, not going near spiders, thinking about something else)

What would be the worst thing that would happen if you came face to face with your fear but could not escape or do the things above? (For example, pass out, die, go crazy, scream and shout, get laughed at)

Home Activity 9a: Hidden worries

Many people find it difficult to think of things that they are afraid of. That's because we usually don't admit to ourselves that we're scared. We say 'I know my limits' and 'I don't see the point', or 'I don't want to' and 'Why should I?'. We stop doing things that make us feel scared because feeling scared is uncomfortable. Make cool connections by looking at things you avoid doing and ask yourself, 'Is it actually because I'm afraid?' Here are some examples:

KATIE: 'I don't want to go to the party. It's not cool' (I'm also scared of being laughed at because I can't find any nice clothes to wear. They all make me look fat and ugly).

HARRY: 'I don't want to play football on the field today – it's boring' (actually I'm frightened there may be a snake lurking in the long grass).

LAUREN: 'I don't want to play in the tennis match – I'm too tired' (and also I'm scared I will let my partner and the team down if I don't play well).

JACK: 'It's too late for you to come to my house for supper' (I'm also scared my parents will be arguing again and that would be embarrassing).

Adapted from Alexander, J. (2006) *Bullies, Bigmouths and So-called Friends.* London: Hodder Children's Books. Text copyright © Jenny Alexander 2003. Reproduced and adapted by permission of Hodder and Stoughton Limited.

Write some things you don't like doing in the box below. Circle the things you avoid doing because of fear.

Home Activity 9b: What do I do?

Think of a time that you felt really afraid, worried or panicky. Complete the boxes below:

What happened? _

_ _

Feelings

Thoughts		**Body signals**

List the things that you did (safety seeking actions) to reduce your worries and calm yourself down. For example, run away, stay at home, etc.

1. _

2. _

3. _

If there is anything you could do differently to help you face your fear next time, write it in the box below:

SESSION 10: Facing Your Fears

Aims and objectives

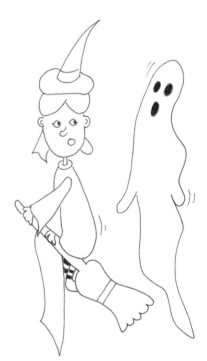

- Learn how to break your problems into smaller, more achievable steps.
- Show how imagining yourself achieving your goals can be helpful.
- Show how modelling yourself on someone who copes well can help you overcome your fears.

Materials

Chairs, pencils, shoe with a lace.

Agenda and tips for running the session

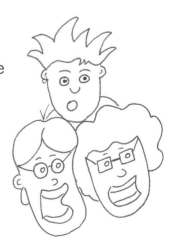

Exercises in bold in the left-hand column should be included in both long and short sessions. Other exercises are optional and can be included in groups where there is more time. Many fun activities/games are included as optional. Despite sometimes being short of time it is important not to cut all the 'fun' out of the programme or you will lose the children's enthusiasm.

Short session

EXERCISE	COMMENTS
Feedback	Welcome the children and share agenda for session with group. Obtain brief feedback from children's week.
Review Home Activities 9a and 9b	Children can briefly discuss their home activities. Facilitators collect home activities to explore in more detail after the session and return the following week or at the end of the programme.
One two I can lace my shoe	Give children two minutes to complete the exercise. Compare the number of steps children have identified. Choose a volunteer to pretend to be an alien and see if he or she can carry out the steps. Unless the steps are broken down clearly it is unlikely that the instructions can be followed.
Feel the fear	Read page 189 to the children and conduct the 'pink elephants theory' in the session. This exercise will illustrate that the harder you avoid or push away 'scary thoughts' the more frightening they become and the more difficult they are to overcome. This exercise is also closely linked with the safety seeking actions described in Session 9.
Cutting your fear down	Illustrates how a fear can develop and be overcome. Children can be asked to volunteer their own experiences of overcoming fears. How did they do it? Who helped them? How do they feel about the fear now?
Step by step	Read through the steps Miss Muffet took to overcome her fear of spiders.

My step plan	Children are encouraged to be specific about what they want to achieve (their goal) and write this at the top of their step plan (step 7). Having identified this goal they can either start at step 1 and work up in small steps or work backwards from their goal at step 7. Children are then encouraged to share their step plans with the group. If children cannot identify a specific fear they can make up a step plan that would help a friend or relative. Learning the process is the important thing in this exercise. If they understand the basic concepts then they can apply the principles to their own fears/difficulties when they are ready.
Home Activity 10a: Imagine, imagine, imagine	The exercise is aimed at helping children visualize themselves coming to terms with their fears. Many people are so avoidant of their fears that simply imagining the fear is a huge step towards coping. For children to visualize themselves just being with their fear can be very empowering and can help boost their confidence.
Home Activity 10b: How we face our fears	This encourages children to work together to generate new ways of coping.

Long session

Include 'One two I can lace my shoe'. Children can be asked to write a short story or draw a picture about a fear. They can create a character and write/ draw about how they overcame the fear using some of the skills they have learned (green light thoughts, visualizing themselves coping, breaking the fear into small steps, etc.). Alternatively, children can act out their step plans with a partner and show the rest of the group.

One two I can lace my shoe

Imagine you have met an alien. He wants you to teach him how to tie his shoe laces. As the alien has never worn shoes before and he does not understand things like 'make a bow' or 'just thread it through there', you are going to have to break your instructions into very small steps and be very clear so that he can understand. List your instructions in the box below. See who in your group can list the most number of steps.

Give your list to a friend and see if they can follow the steps if they do exactly what your instructions say.

Lace my shoe: instructions for an alien

Feel the fear

Most people who have a fear or worry try to avoid it at all costs. They don't want to hear about it, think about it or talk about it, and most of all they don't want to have to face it. They just want it to go away. The trouble is that worries don't always just go away. In fact sometimes the more you try to avoid or not think about your worries the more they seem to bug you.

Pink elephants theory

As an example of this, close your eyes and try really hard not to think about pink elephants. What happened? Most people find that they think about pink elephants. This goes to show that the more you try not to think about something the worse it becomes.

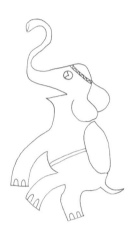

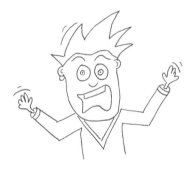

The truth is that the only real way to completely get rid of your worries is to face up to them. Like the saying goes, 'Feel the fear and do it anyway' (Jeffers 1987).

This is easier said than done but some ideas that might help you include:

- Thinking green light thoughts (see Session 7).

- Take small steps.

- Imagine yourself achieving your goals or coping with your problem or fear.

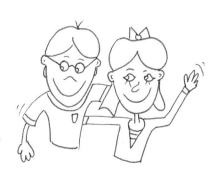

Reference: Jeffers, S. (1987) *Feel the fear and Do It Anyway: How to Turn Your Fear and Indecision into Confidence and Action.* Ballantine Books

Cutting your fear down

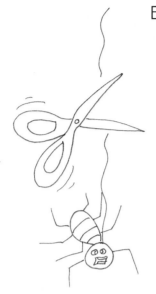

Everyone knows that if you fall off a horse you should get back in the saddle as soon as possible. That's because when you've had a bad experience you fear it could happen again, and the sooner you face up to the fear the easier it is to get over it. The longer you put off facing up to fear, the bigger it grows. By the time the fear's got bigger than you, there's no way you can tackle it head on. You have to work up to it in stages, starting with smaller fears first.

Extract from Alexander, J. (2006) *Bullies, Bigmouths and So-called Friends.* London: Hodder Children's Books. Text copyright © Jenny Alexander 2003. Reproduced and adapted by permission of Hodder and Stoughton Limited

Lauren's high dive

Lauren has been having diving coaching at the local swimming pool. She really enjoys it and is doing well. She can do lots of different dives. She can go backwards and she can even do a somersault into the water. The trouble is that since she did a belly flop a few years ago she has become too afraid to dive from the top board. Her parents have offered her a present if she can pluck up the courage but it just seems too high. When Lauren looks down from the edge of the high board her legs feel like jelly and her knees knock together. She thinks to herself, 'It's just too scary. I'm sure to hurt myself.' Frightening pictures flash through her head of belly flops, people laughing at her and hospitals. Poor Lauren believes that she will never learn to dive from the top board.

Lauren's coach does not despair. He patiently encourages her to practise an easy dive over and over again from the side of the swimming pool. Gradually she progresses from the poolside on to the first board. Lauren uses a step-by-step approach to face her fear. After perfecting the first diving board Lauren's coach encourages her to go higher and dive from the second board. Although she is a little nervous to begin with she quickly gains confidence and dives beautifully. She even completes a few somersaults to show off her skills to her mum and dad who are watching in the swimming pool gallery. Eventually Lauren's coach suggests she try from the top. Nervously Lauren stands on the end of the board. It does not seem so high this time, after all her practice. Having pictured herself doing the dive successfully in her mind as her coach instructed, Lauren raises her arms, then pauses for a moment before jumping high into the air. She felt the wind rush through her hair and her body whizz round as she completed the dive and plunged through the water perfectly. Success. She had done it. Her parents and coach clapped as she rushed up the steps of the diving board with excitement to do it all over again. Lauren had taken small steps and overcome her fear.

Can you think of a time when you overcame a fear like Lauren in the example above? How did you cut your fear down to size?

Step by step

In order to face something that you are afraid of it can be helpful to break the fear into small steps. In the example below make cool connections by seeing how Little Miss Muffet overcomes her fear of spiders using a step-by-step approach. You do not have to be afraid of spiders to use this approach. In fact this same approach can be used to overcome any fear from heights, water, insects, mice, talking in public, sickness or school. The most important thing is to start with your goal in step 7. This should contain what you want to be able to do when you have overcome your fear. Note that Little Miss Muffet does not have to like spiders to get over her fear. She is satisfied just to have one walk on her hand.

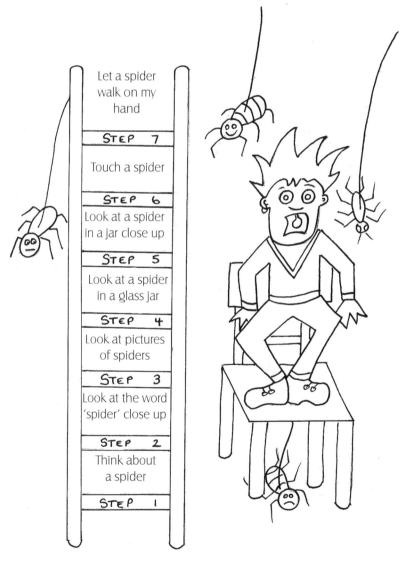

My step plan

As no two people are the same, everyone's step-by-step ladder will be different. To begin, write your goal at the top of your ladder (step 7). Following this, complete steps 1 to 6 with step 1 as the easiest step and the rest getting more difficult. The smaller the steps the more likely you are to achieve your goal.

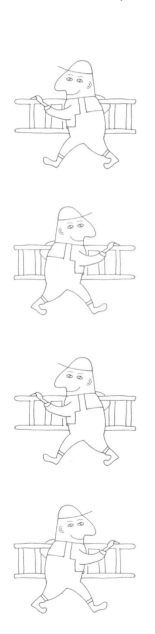
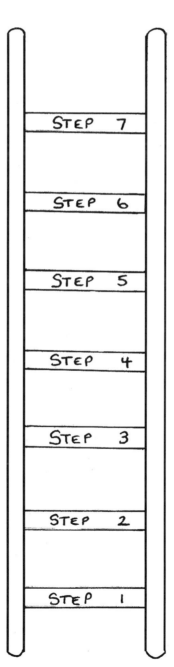
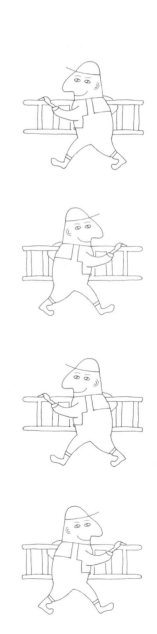

Home Activity 10a: Imagine, imagine, imagine

To overcome problems or fears it can be very helpful to imagine yourself coping. Let your mind go wild and dream up some cool ways to overcome your fears. Use magic to turn the bullies into frogs, dive from the top diving board, get an A in your science test, imagine super powers to cope with frightening monsters. Whatever, make sure you come out on top. Either draw or use modelling materials to create your scene. Share your ideas with the group.

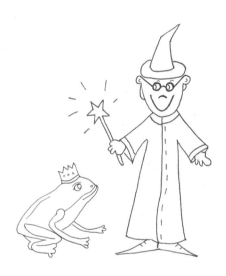

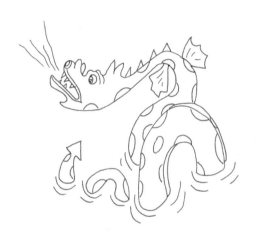

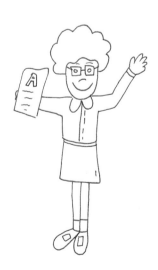

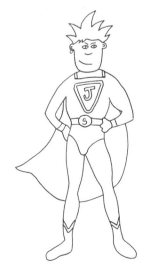

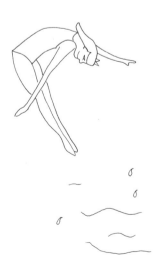

Home Activity 10b: How we face our fears

Get together with a friend from the group during the week. Design a poster, or make a little show, dance or pop song, to demonstrate how you made cool connections to face your fears. Performances will take place next session and should last no longer than three minutes each. Try to include as many of the following ways of coping in your presentation:

- taking small steps
- imagine yourself coping
- thinking of how a good 'coper' could tackle your fears
- thinking green light thoughts.

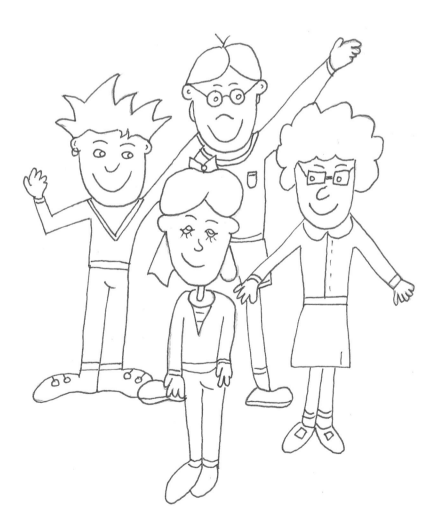

Evaluation

Aims and objectives

- Evaluate the programme.
- Find out what we have learned.
- See if the group has helped with your feelings.
- Find some ideas on how to improve the group for other children in the future.
- Congratulate each other on completing the programme and receive a certificate.

Materials

Chairs, pencils.

Agenda and tips for running the session

Exercises in bold in the left-hand column should be included in both long and short sessions. Many fun activities/games are included as optional. Despite sometimes being short of time it is important not to cut all the 'fun' out of the programme or you will lose the children's enthusiasm.

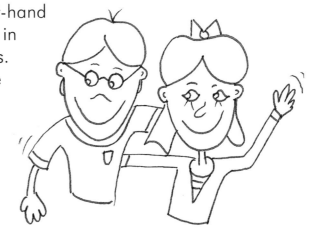

Short session

EXERCISE	COMMENTS
Feedback	Welcome the children and share agenda for session with group. Obtain brief feedback from children's week.
Review Home Activities 10a and 10b	Children can share and discuss their home activities. Children are encouraged to show or perform their home activity in front of the group.
Game	Children are invited to choose one or two of the games played in sessions earlier in the programme.
Re-rate yourself	Children are encouraged to re-rate themselves. Compare the ratings with the same exercise on page 53 in Session 1. It is useful to discuss with the children what they make of any changes that have taken place. What have they learned/experienced to contribute to the change in the rating scores?
Cool connections evaluation	Children complete the cool connections evaluation. The first seven questions reflect the basic aims and objectives of the programme. Children are encouraged to add any further comments if they wish.

Long session

You may wish to include a mini party as a celebration for completing the programme. This could include cakes, drinks, etc. You may wish to make your own certificates and present them to the children.

Notes

In some cases when the children re-rate themselves, the level of fear or upset may appear to have got worse since the beginning of the programme. This does not matter. It is only a measure. It is possible that a child's personal/ environmental circumstances may have changed to influence their feelings. For example, during the programme they may have experienced a significant loss or trauma. Some children have also reported that as the programme progressed they learned more about their feelings and were better able to give an accurate measure of their feelings by the end of the programme. This indicates that the measures recorded at the beginning of the programme were inaccurate.

Re-rate yourself

Mark a cross on the number you currently feel most represents your life and how you are coping both in and out of school.

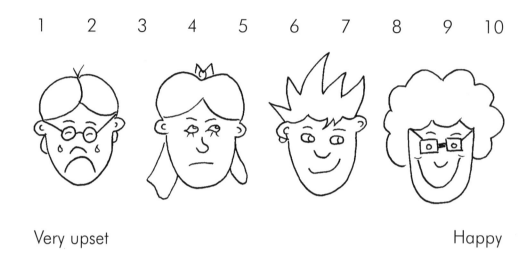

| 1 | 2 | 3 | 4 | 5 | 6 | 7 | 8 | 9 | 10 |

Very upset   Happy

List the three things below which you felt most upset about in your life at the beginning of the programme. (You may need to refer back to p.53) Put a cross on the number which best represents how you feel now.

Example: ___ I have not got many friends _____

1   2   3   4   5   6   7   8   9̶   10
Very upset   Happy

1. _____

1   2   3   4   5   6   7   8   9   10
Very upset   Happy

2. _____

1   2   3   4   5   6   7   8   9   10
Very upset   Happy

3. _____

1   2   3   4   5   6   7   8   9   10
Very upset   Happy

Cool connections evaluation

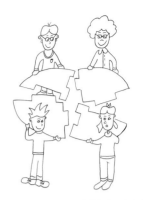

For each of the following questions please put a tick in the boxes below.

Have you had fun in the group?

Not at all	A little bit	A lot	Loads

Has being in the group helped you get on better with other children?

Not at all	A little bit	A lot	Very much

Has being in the group helped you feel more confident?

Not at all	A little bit	A lot	Very much

Has being in the group given you new experiences?

Not at all	A little bit	A lot	Loads

Do you think that the group has helped you feel better about yourself?

Not at all	A little bit	A lot	Very much

Has being in the group helped you with your worries?

Not at all	A little bit	A lot	Very much

What would you tell other children about the Cool Connections group?

Load of rubbish	They were OK	Very good	Super cool and brilliant

Further comments about the group:

Self-Esteem Games for Children

Deborah M. Plummer
Illustrations by Jane Serrurier

Paperback, ISBN 978 1 84310 424 7, 144 pages

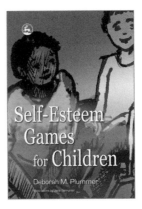

'The book contains so many fresh ideas for group therapy; readers will be inspired and well-equipped to promote self-esteem more often in practice. It is excellent value for money.'

– Speech and Language Therapy in Practice

In this practical handbook, self-esteem expert Deborah Plummer offers a wealth of familiar and easy-to-learn games carefully chosen to build and maintain self-esteem in children aged 5–11.

The selection of games reflects the seven key elements of healthy self-esteem – self-knowledge, self and others, self-acceptance, self-reliance, self-expression, self-confidence and self-awareness – and includes opportunities for thinking and discussion. The book combines physically active and passive games, verbal and non-verbal games and games for pairs or groups, which makes them equally accessible for children with speech/language difficulties or those with physical disabilities. Deborah Plummer shows that the games can be easily adapted and she encourages readers to be creative in inventing their own alternative versions.

This is an ideal resource for teachers, parents, carers and all those working to nurture self-esteem in children.

Deborah Plummer is a registered speech and language therapist and imagework practitioner with over 20 years' experience of facilitating groups and working individually with both children and adults. She is a clinical supervisor and lecturer and runs workshops and short courses on the uses of imagery and issues of self-esteem in the UK and abroad.

Helping Children to Build Self-Esteem

A Photocopiable Activities Book

Second Edition

Deborah M. Plummer
Illustrations by Alice Harper

Paperback, ISBN 978 1 84310 488 9, 288 pages

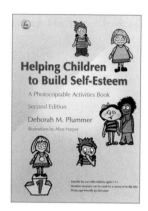

'An excellent resource that teaches ways of helping every child to build self esteem. I recommend it wholeheartedly to parents, childminders and professional childcare providers.'

– National Childminding Association, www.nmca.org.uk'

This second edition of the highly successful *Helping Children to Build Self-Esteem* is packed with fun and effective activities to help children develop and maintain healthy self-esteem.

New and updated material has been added including a section on running parent groups alongside children's groups, as well as a brand new layout, fresh illustrations, an expanded theoretical section and extra activities.

Based on the author's extensive clinical experience, this activities book will equip and support teaching staff, therapists and carers in encouraging feelings of competence and self-worth in children and their families. It is primarily designed for use with individuals and groups of children aged 7–11, but the ideas can easily be adapted for both older and younger children and children with learning difficulties.

This fully photocopiable resource is invaluable for anyone looking for creative, practical ways of nurturing self-esteem in children.

Helping Adolescents and Adults to Build Self-Esteem

A Photocopiable Book

Deborah M. Plummer

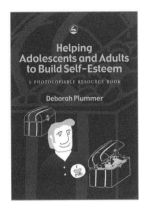

Paperback, ISBN 978 1 84310 185 7, 272 pages

'The book is practical, positive and easy to use and is an invaluable resource for anyone looking for positive, practical ways of nurturing confidence and self-esteem.'

– NAGC Magazine

A healthy level of individual self-esteem is the foundation for emotional, physical and social well-being. People who value themselves and who recognise their own skills are likely to live fulfilling and rewarding lives and will tend to attract genuine liking and respect from others. Conversely, low levels of self-esteem have been linked with such personal and social concerns as school failure, depression, social anxiety, violence and substance abuse.

Helping Adolescents and Adults to Build Self-Esteem follows on from the widely acclaimed *Helping Children to Build Self-Esteem*. It is filled with simple, practical and innovative ideas for supporting the development and maintenance of healthy self-esteem. Based on the author's clinical experience, the easy-to-use photocopiable activity sheets encourage participants to draw on existing skills and to develop new approaches to building confidence and feelings of self-worth. These exercises are suitable for work with individuals and with groups, and will prove an indispensable aid to building self-esteem in adolescents and adults.

Anger Management Games for Children

Deborah M. Plummer
Illustrations by Jane Serrurier

Paperback, ISBN 978 1 84310 628 9, 160 pages

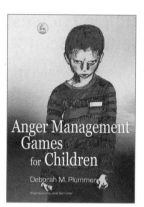

This practical handbook helps adults to understand, manage and reflect constructively on children's anger. Featuring a wealth of familiar and easy-to-learn games, it is designed to foster successful anger management strategies for children aged 5–12.

The book covers the theory behind the games in accessible language, and includes a broad range of enjoyable activities: active and passive, verbal and non-verbal, and for different sized groups. The games address issues that might arise in age-specific situations such as sharing a toy or facing peer pressure. They also encourage children to approach their emotions as a way to facilitate personal growth and healthy relationships.

This is an ideal resource for teachers, parents, carers and all those working with anger management in children.

No More Stinking Thinking

A Workbook for Teaching Children Positive Thinking

Joann Altiero

Paperback, ISBN 978 1 84310 839 9, 60 pages

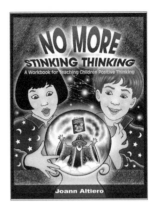

'This ingenious workbook, designed for use by psychologists, teachers or parents, is highly visual and interactive and could beneficially be used with individuals and groups of children.'

– *The Psychologist*

How can children learn to combat negative thinking in a fun and constructive way? By applying to be a wizard of positive thinking, of course!

Joann Altiero's *No More Stinking Thinking* is an easy-to-use workbook for use by parents, teachers, and therapists to teach children how to develop the cognitive skills and resilience that will help them to cope with daily adversity, including criticism, disappointment and bullying. Each lesson in this mental health "wizard class" explains a different type of "Stinking Thinking" – from ignoring the big picture or jumping to conclusions to making a big (or little) deal out of something – and teaches children how to spot and combat it. They are drawn into a magical world where they learn about the power of positive, healthy and confident thinking and assertive behaviors as they defeat the evil Lord Stinker and become "Super Thinking Wizards." Exercises, a final "exam," and a graduation certificate are included.

Accessible and fully interactive, *No More Stinking Thinking* is an ideal tool for helping children develop positive thinking skills in an imaginative and exciting way.

Joann Altiero, Ph.D., is a child clinical psychologist who received her doctorate from Southern Illinois University. She has worked in the field of clinical psychology for over 20 years, is a faculty member at the University of Maryland University College and has had a successful private practice promoting family mental health in La Plata, MD, since 1998.

The Complete Guide to Asperger's Syndrome

Tony Attwood

Hardback, ISBN 978 1 84310 495 7, 400 pages
Paperback, ISBN 978 1 84310 669 2, 400 pages

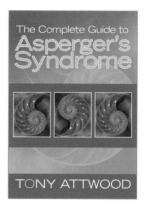

'A comprehensive manual filled with useful information, updated research and most importantly, helpful advice and encouragement for those of us who have AS and those who strive to support us.'

– Liane Holliday Willey, EdD
author of Pretending to be Normal: Living With Asperger's Syndrome

The Complete Guide to Asperger's Syndrome is the definitive handbook for anyone affected by Asperger's syndrome (AS). It brings together a wealth of information on all aspects of the syndrome for children through to adults.

Drawing on case studies and personal accounts from Attwood's extensive clinical experience, and from his correspondence with individuals with AS, this book is both authoritative and extremely accessible. Chapters examine:

- causes and indications of the syndrom
- the diagnosis and its effect on the individual
- theory of mind
- the perception of emotions in self and others
- social interaction, including friendships
- long-term relationships
- teasing, bullying and mental health issues
- the effect of AS on language and cognitive abilities, sensory sensitivity, movement and co-ordination skills
- career development.

There is also an invaluable frequently asked questions chapter and a section listing useful resources for anyone wishing to find further information on a particular aspect of AS, as well as literature and educational tools.

Essential reading for families and individuals affected by AS as well as teachers, professionals and employers coming in contact with people with AS, this book should be on the bookshelf of anyone who needs to know or is interested in this complex condition.

Tony Attwood is a practising clinical psychologist with more than 25 years' experience. He has worked with over 2000 individuals of all ages with Asperger's syndrome. He presents workshops and runs training courses for parents, professionals and individuals with AS all over the world and is a prolific author of articles and books on the subject.